ATHLETIC BODY TRAINING

ATHLETIC BODY TRAINING

Over 140 Bodyweight, Jump Rope, and Sandbag exercises to Develop your Athleticism

TRACEY E. BAILEY

LIBRARY OF CONGRESS CONTROL NUMBER: 2010908200
ISBN: HARDCOVER   978-1-4535-1679-9
                      SOFTCOVER   978-1-4535-1678-2

No book or video can replace the services of a trained doctor, exercise physiologist, and or qualified fitness professional. Applying the information in this publication is at the reader's risk and discretion.

Credits

Photographers—Tracey Bailey and select photos by Aldonia Bailey
Assistant photographers—Jessica Bailey, Angel Bailey
Photo Editor—Tracey Bailey
Models—Tracey Bailey, Nigel Bailey, Byron Bailey, Steve S., Bryan Streit

This book was printed in the United States of America.

To order additional copies of this book, contact:
Xlibris Corporation
1-888-795-4274
www.Xlibris.com
Orders@Xlibris.com
68440

CONTENTS

This book is dedicated to my family, my wife Jessica, I could not have completed this book without you, my daughters, Aubrey and Autumn and, my son Malik, I love you.

Preface

Will I get results from the exercises and workouts in this book?

Yes. If you work hard training with the exercises in this book or implement the routines into your workouts, you can count on getting results. But beware, you might attain results to the extent of being accused of spending too much time in the gym or too much money on supplements.

Consistency is the key.

You will get results from the exercises and workouts in this book by using them on a consistent bases. I recommend safely attempting a routine at least twice a week; try adding or substituting a few exercise movements to challenge yourself. Keep in mind that the key to your athletic body fitness level is consistency, so you have stick to it.

Are the exercises new?

I've been asked a couple of times, are your exercises new? I thought they were, but human movement is not new. In fact, there is nothing new under the sun, just old stuff rediscovered. Things like push-ups, pull-ups, running with weights, and weighed backpacks, climbing up a doorway like Spiderman, doing dips between the kitchen counters or on a rehab walker is not new. I've been doing them since I was eight years old.

Who should use the exercises in this book?

The exercises in this book are for everyone because there are exercises for every fitness level. Having sufficient strength, coordination, and balance are required for some of the exercises. If you cannot perform a certain exercise with the proper technique, try selecting another exercise within the same category. You can also try modifying the exercise. Although modifying the exercise might not allow you to attain the full benefit of the exercise, with safe practice, getting the results you want should be right around the corner.

Acknowledgement

I would like to thank all of the athletes, coaches, clients and, health care professionals that I've been privileged to work with over the past 12 years. I also gratefully thank all of the following for helping me harness my energy and focus to strive to do all that I can to help others; thank you: Jehovah, thank you for everything. Angel Bailey, Byron Bailey, Crystal Bailey, Yolanda Bailey, Aldonia Bailey, Alvin Bailey Jr., Darren Bailey, and, Greylin Bailey. A special thank you to all of your sons and daughters especially Nigel Bailey who overcame many physical obstacles. Steve S., Bryan Streit, Dr Alex Baek, Ok Bon Han, Dr Richard Sayegh, Dr Harry Wurmsdobler, Dr. Mike, Coach Bob Takano—takanoathletics.com, Coach Mike Burgener, Mark Haro, Margie Seitz, Rick Krost. To the following people who have a had a positive impact on my life, Mckinnis family, Steve Cha, Eddie, Linda and Melissa Temple, Patricia Ernst, Jim Defrisco, GeorgeYasmin, Bob Martin, Ted, Shirl and Curtis Sams, Spencer Hill, Carrie Lenard, Roger Sanchez and family. Thank all of you for the good that you have done for me and many other people. Keep up the good work!

Chapter 1

BODY WEIGHT TRAINING

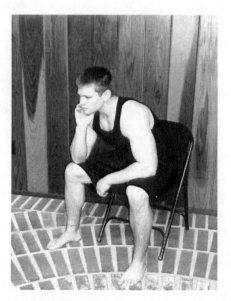

WHY BODY WEIGHT TRAINING?

For many years, people have been using their own body weight to gain strength and to condition the body. From learning to crawl as a toddler to climbing up a mountain, moving your own body weight has always and will always be the key to health and fitness. Ask yourself, how can a person be healthy and strong if they cannot get up as many times as they need to? Consider this, what if you could not stand up without using your arms to assist you? What if you did not have the strength to pull yourself up, push yourself up, or simply sit up with ease? Would you feel healthy and strong? Then ask yourself, can I perform pull-ups, push-ups, and squats? If not, am I really healthy and fit?

The point is being able to move ourselves, is where true health and fitness is at today, and every day. Being able to easily move ourselves is something else.

BODY CONTROL

What do you think of when you think of body control? Some think of being able to control their body while moving at slow or top speeds in any safe anatomical position and in any given direction. Yes, that sounds correct, but what about moving on your hands? Although your sport or lifestyle might not require you to move on your hands, having the ability to do so would enhance your body control and improve your entire fitness level.

Although some people are content with their body control—including getting up, getting in the car as part of their fitness routine on the way to the gym, to hop on a couple of machines, tease the abs, and top off the routine with some cardio—others want more and get more with less time.

BODY AWARENESS

Body awareness, also known as kinetic awareness, is not limited to being aware of how our arms, legs, back, shoulders, abs, and chest muscles move. It also involves being able to coordinate the timing, speed, and rhythm of a movement or movements as well.

Using our own body's weight to exercise couldn't be beat by another fitness tool. Besides, lifting an object starts by moving a body part; case closed, end of argument. Being able to move and control your body's own weight, will allow you the potential to involve your core in almost every exercise; therefore, you will become more in tune with your central nervous system. You will notice the results by your having more body control with every limb in all positions.

Body weight training is also very effective in developing isometric strength in the primary muscles as well as the muscles stabilizing the movements. Many people that have performed body weight exercises like push-ups have said, there're too easy because they were use to performing them. They are correct.

Fortunately, while in training, I was able to help them understand how easy and strenuous push-ups can really be. When you perform some of the exercises you will notice you will need a sufficient amount of strength, coordination, and balance for some of the exercises. If you cannot perform a certain exercise with the proper technique, try selecting another exercise within the same category. If the exercise is too easy, then select one that is more challenging. The clients that received firsthand push-up variations during a session with me gained tremendous results. We would train with the "easy" push-ups to fatigue, then move on to using a dive bomber push-up to one-leg push-ups to incline dive bomber push-ups to failure. Changing the angle and or the type of movement gave them exactly what they were looking for.

Over the years of training a variety of people with a variety of goals, I've learned many things. The one thing that stood out the most was, not everyone wants to train to failure even if they agree to and or need to train to failure to reach there goals. The cause of their resistance is DOMS or delayed onset muscle soreness a.k.a. lactic acid *soreness*.

One key to getting results from any training program is adaptability. DOMS is primarily caused by forces placed on the eccentric muscle contractions (e.g., the downward phase of a movement) during exercise. Our bodies will need consistent training to build up a tolerance for the lactic acid and to train at a high level.

A benefit of training at a high level is one, results, and two, the positive effects it has on our internal organs. That's why training to failure isn't all bad. Not only does the muscle get in shape, but several adapting hormonal responses are required to build up a high exercise tolerance. To name a few, if done correctly, our heart, lungs, kidney, and liver also get in shape.

BODY WEIGHT EXERCISES ARE SAFE

The average person can probably strain a muscle on a bench press by using too much weight or working out with poor form or both. But if you get tired while performing a push-up, you won't have to worry about the weights falling on you. Generally, if you cannot perform another push-up, your body won't move, which should give you enough time to safely stop, rest, or move on. The majority of the people that I've worked with have benefited by starting out using body weight or implementing body weight exercises into an advanced routine.

SUMMARY

There is overwhelming support and evidence that point to body weight exercises as an excellent way to develop an athletic body and fitness for everyone. The problem is knowing what to do and how to move. The following chapter will assist you by illustrating exercises to use and add to your workouts.

Chapter 2

Body Weight Exercises

Core Exercises

Core Exercises are exercises that require using one or more large muscle(s) in an exercise, along with using several muscles that recruit one primary joint. I like to consider the subsequent core exercises as whole-body, multi-joint movements and placed them in the book for your health and athletic development.

This section of the book will provide you with a variety of exercises you can use on a daily or weekly basis or to supplement your own workouts.

Body Weight Core Exercises

Wheelbarrow

Beginning Position:
Start with feet on a stability ball/medicine ball or have a partner hold your feet.

Action:
With your hands on the floor and your body in push-up position, keep your abs, glutes, and back tight.
Walk out in a given direction and distance.

Optional: Alternate your legs as you walk on your hands.

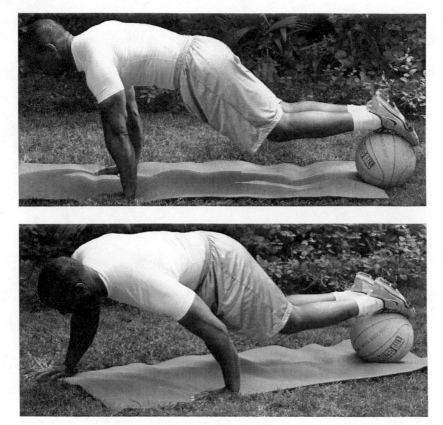

Photo by Aldonia Bailey

BODY WEIGHT CORE EXERCISES

3-D Up Down

Beginning Position:
Start while in push-up position.

Action:

1. Keep your hands on the floor. Hop to your right or left side and slightly tuck your legs in. Keep your hands on the floor to hop and return to the center starting push-up position.

2. From the center starting push-up position, hands still on the floor, hop and tuck your legs into your chest. Return to the center starting push-up position.

3. From the center starting push-up position, hop to the opposite side of step 1, and slightly tuck your legs in and return to the center starting push-up position.

4. From the center starting push-up position, hop and land in a deep squat position with your feet flat and shoulder-width apart.

Ending Position:
From the squat position, jump up, land on your feet, and hop back into the push-up position to repeat the exercise

Optional Variation:
1. Perform one push-up after steps 1-3.
2. Perform a push-up every time you center yourself into the starting push-up position.
3. Alternate your starting side after each up down.

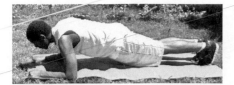

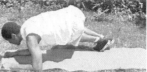

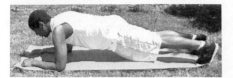

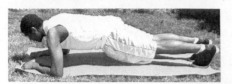

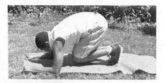

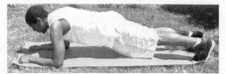

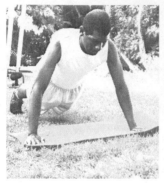

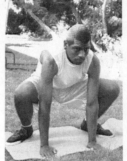

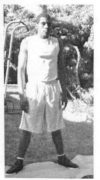

BODY WEIGHT CORE EXERCISES

Floor Windmill

Beginning Position:
While in push-up position, place your hands directly under your sternum.

Action:
Stabilize your body weight on one hand and rotate into a straight-arm side plank. Continue rotating until you place your other hand on the floor.

Note:
Try to keep your hands under your deltoids when you're in the supine/chest-up position.

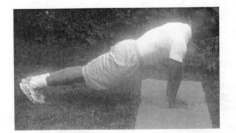

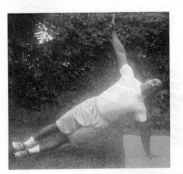

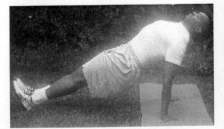

Photo by Aldonia Bailey

BODY WEIGHT CORE EXERCISES

Standing Windmill

Beginning Position:
Stand with your feet shoulder-width apart. Allow yourself to fall back on one arm while keeping your hips up with a straight back.

Action:
Use your leg, hips, and abs to bounce up as you rotate your upper body to relax and fall back to touch the floor with your other hand.

Note: Keep your arms aligned with your shoulder.

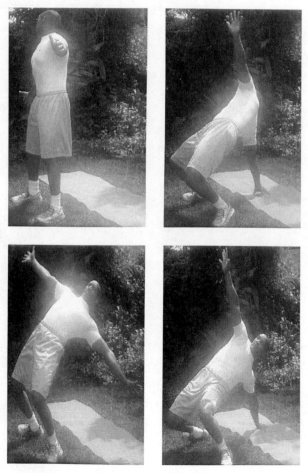

Photo by Aldonia Bailey

BODY WEIGHT CORE EXERCISE

Hand Walks

Beginning Position:
Sit on your feet with your hands on the floor.

Action:
Tuck your legs and knees up to your chest and walk with your hands. Feel free to cover your legs under your shirt.

Note: try to walk sideways.

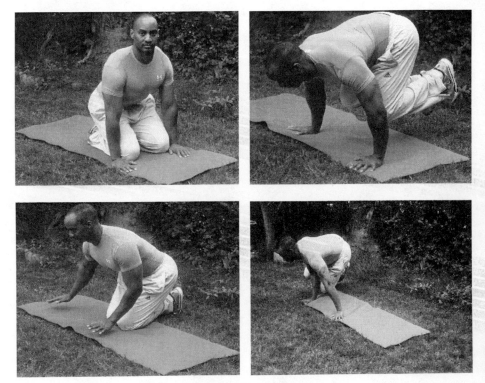

Photo by Aldonia Bailey

Body Weight Core Exercises

Bear Crawl

Beginning Position:
Start with both hands and feet on the floor, keep your hips elevated while keeping your chest low to the ground.

Action:
Crawl in the bear position for a distance or for a specific time.

Note: keep your head and neck aligned with your back.

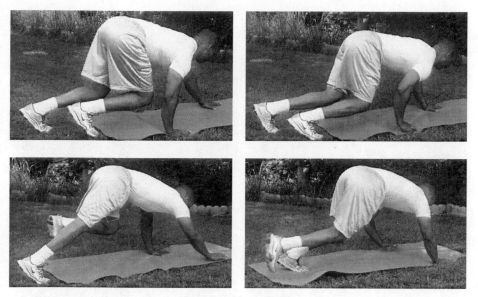

Photo by Aldonia Bailey

BODY WEIGHT CORE EXERCISES

Time Clocks

Beginning Position:
Start while in an elevated push-up position.

Action:
Lift your left or right leg up and swing it until it touches the floor near your hand. Immediately swing your leg back until it touches your other leg. Upon touching your leg, swing your leg to touch near your hand, and return your leg toward your other side to repeat the movement

Note:
Try to mimic a grandfather clock.

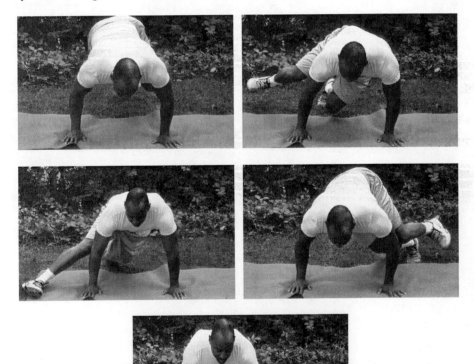

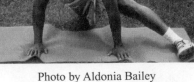

Photo by Aldonia Bailey

BODY WEIGHT CORE EXERCISE

Time Clock Burpee

Beginning Position:
Perform a time clock exercise.

Action:
After each rep, you should be in the push-up position. While in the push-up position, hop your feet forward to get into the squat position and stand or jump up.

Optional:
When you're in the push-up position, perform a push-up before you stand or jump up.

BODY WEIGHT CORE EXERCISES

Up Down/Burpee

Beginning Position:
Stand with your feet shoulder-width apart.

Action:
Squat down and place your hands on the floor, about shoulder-width apart. Hop back with your legs to place yourself into push-up position.

Hop your feet forward into the squat position and stand up or jump up.

Optional:
When you're in the push-up position, perform an upper body pushing exercise.

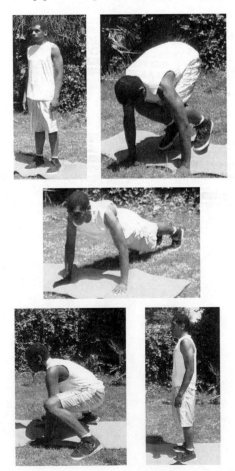

BODY WEIGHT CORE EXERCISES

Up Down
Grasshopper Burpee

Beginning Position:
Start in a push-up position, with your hands on the floor, lift your right or left leg.

Action:
Rotate your waist after your leg is past your waist and chest. Return your leg to the beginning position and repeat the movement with your other leg without pausing. Return to the push-up position to complete the movement by jumping up into the burpee.

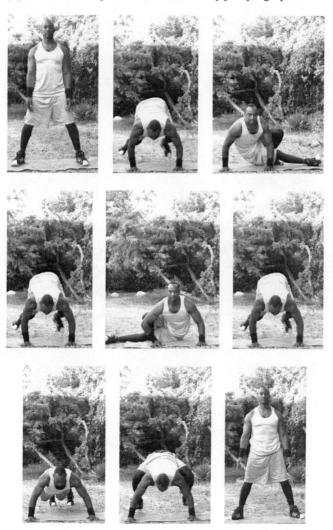

CORE BODY WEIGHT EXERCISE

3-D Plank Jump

Beginning Position:
Start while in plank position.

Action:
1. Keep your arms and hands on the floor, hop to your right or left side, and slightly tuck your legs in. Without pausing, hop into a plank then hop into the push up position.

2. Keep your hands on the floor, hop forward to bring your feet toward your hands without pausing. Hop and return to the push up position.

3. Keep your hands on the floor, hop into a plank. Without pausing, hop to your other side and slightly tuck your legs in. Return to the push up position to hop into a squat and jump up.

Picture notes:
Start plank—hop, tuck on one side—return to plank—hop, push up position, feet to hands return to push up position, to plank, hop tuck on the other side, to push up position, to deep squat, and jump.

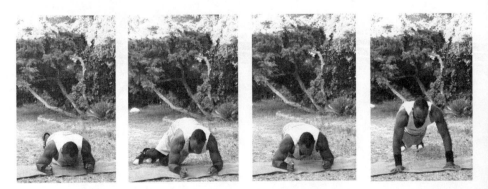

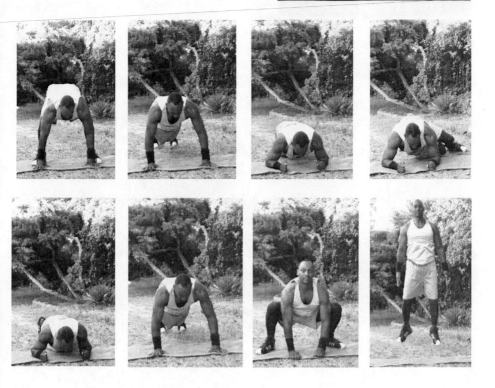

BODY WEIGHT CORE EXERCISES

Side-to-side Squat
Burpee

Beginning Position:
Start with your feet slightly beyond shoulder-width apart.

Action:
Squat down on your left or right side. After you squat down on your left or right side, below ninety-degree flexion at your knees and hips, shift your body weight to the other side. When you have performed the side-to-side squat, return to the beginning position and drop down in push-up position to perform your burpee. When you complete your burpee, return to your standing position for more reps.

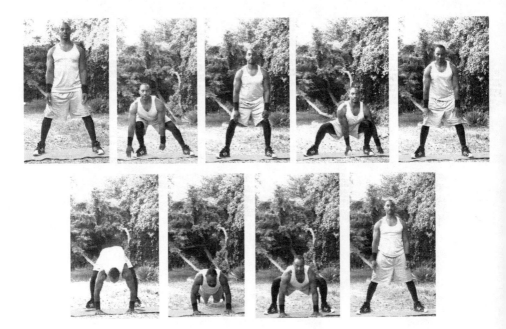

Upper Body Pulling Exercises

Upper Body Pulling Exercise Notes

When performing a standing pull-up type exercise, bend your knees if the bar is not high enough to allow full range of motion.

Modified Pull-up/Chin-up

Beginning Position:
Using a straight bar or dip station.

Action:
Grip the bar(s). While keeping your body, hips, and knees straight, pull yourself up to complete the reps.

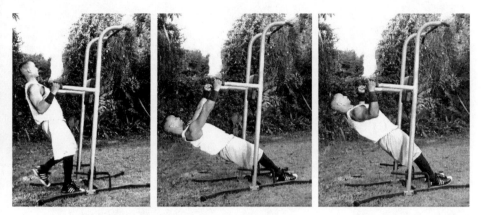

UPPER BODY PULLING EXERCISES

Jumping Pull-up

Beginning Position:
Start while holding your pull-up/chin-up bar.

Action:
Use your legs to jump and elevate yourself by pulling yourself up to complete the exercise.

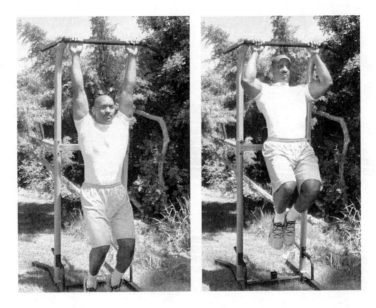

Upper Body Pulling Exercises

Chin-up

Beginning Position:
Place your hands on the bar about five inches away from your shoulders with your palms facing your body.

Action:
Pull yourself up until your chin passes the bar.

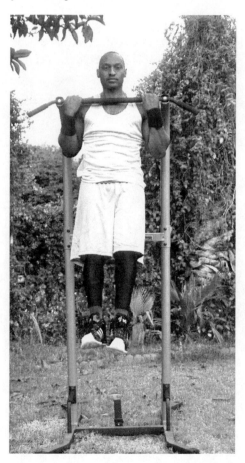

UPPER BODY PULLING EXERCISES

Pull-up

Beginning Position:
Place your palms on the bar about five inches away from your shoulders with your knuckles facing your body.

Action:
Pull yourself up until your chin passes the bar.

Optional
1. Lift your knees above your belly button with every rep to work your abs.
2. Perform every rep with your legs straight by holding them in the air, parallel to the ground.

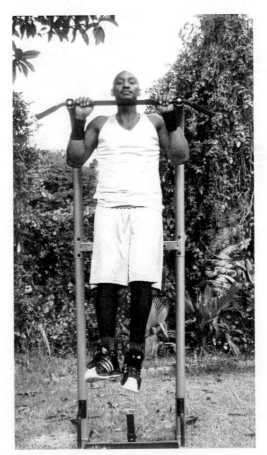

UPPER BODY PULLING EXERCISES

Bicep Blaster

Beginning Position:
Start with your hands on the bar facing your body.

Action:
Perform a chin-up. Lower yourself halfway down and pull yourself up until your chin passes the bar to complete one rep.

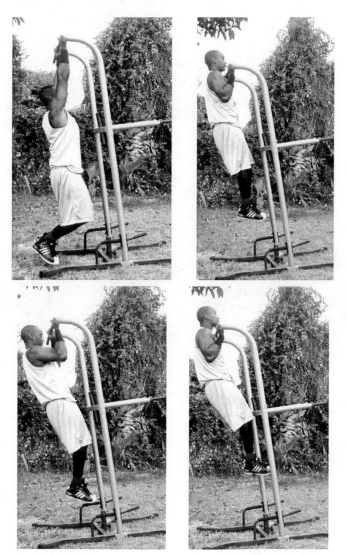

UPPER BODY PULLING EXERCISES

Alternating Pull-up/Chin-up

Beginning Position:
Alternate your grip with both hands on the bar, about five inches away from your shoulders.

Action:
Pull yourself up.

Optional:
After you lower your body, alternate each arm per rep.

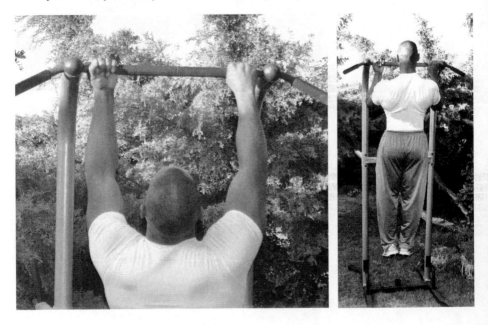

UPPER BODY PULLING EXERCISES

Circle Pull-up/Circle Chin-up

Beginning Position:
Select your grip to perform the pull-up or chin-up method.

Action:
Pull your body up so your arm is in front of the center of your chest as you lower your body. Shift your body weight to your other arm. Pull yourself up using a circular motion.

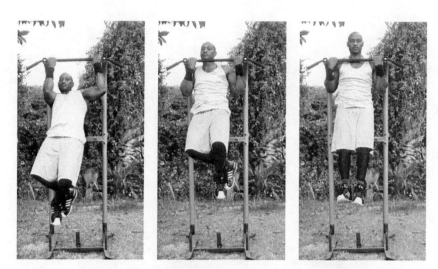

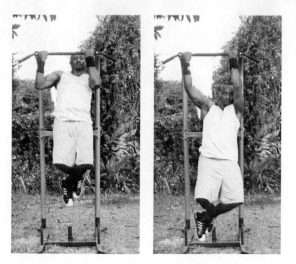

U PPER B ODY P ULLING E XERCISES

Side-to-side Pull-up/Chin-up

Beginning Position:
Select your grip to perform the pull-up or chin-up method.

Action:
Pull yourself up. While holding yourself up, keep your chin over the bar and move your entire body from side to side.

Optional:
Use chin-up grip.

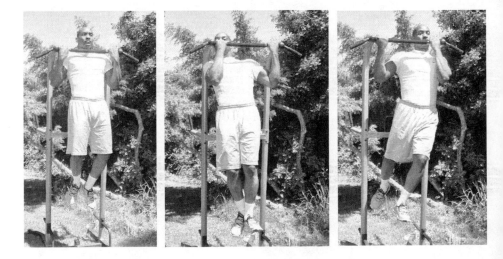

UPPER BODY PULLING EXERCISES

Modified One-arm Pull-up/Chin-up

Beginning Position:
Select your grip for your pulling arm. Use the opposite grip for your support arm.

Action:
Pull your body up using your primary pulling arm while counterbalancing with your support arm.

Note:
Try not to overuse your support arm.

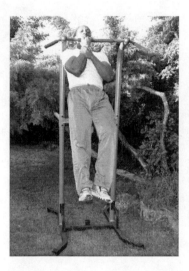 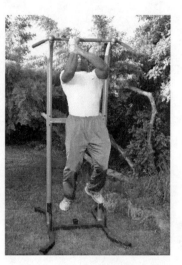

UPPER BODY PULLING EXERCISES

One-arm Pull-up

Beginning Position:
Start while standing in pull-up/chin-up position and holding your bar with one hand, place your nonworking hand at your side or behind your back.

Action:
Pull yourself up with one arm. Perform the same number of pull-ups on both arms.

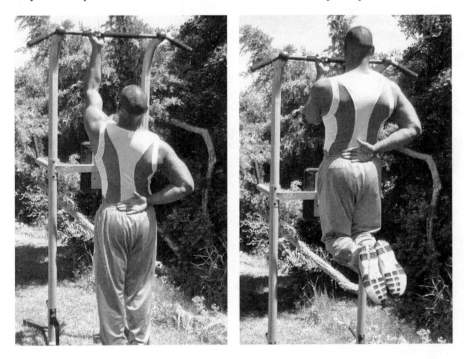

UPPER BODY PULLING EXERCISES

Modified Horizontal Row

Beginning Position:
Start while lying on the floor with your back on the ground, knees bent, and feet flat on the ground, position your elbows eight inches away from your body.

Action:
Keep your glutes on the floor and lift your shoulders and back off the ground by rowing against the floor.

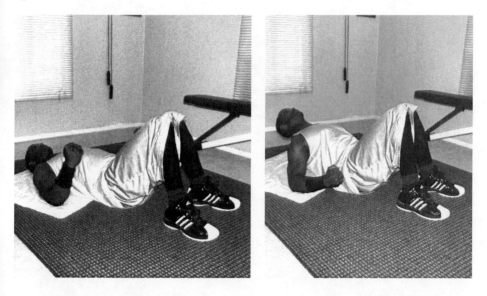

UPPER BODY PULLING EXERCISES

Horizontal Row

Beginning Position:
Start while lying on the floor with your back on the ground, knees bent, and feet flat on the ground, position your elbows eight inches away from your body.

Action:
Lift your shoulders, back, and glutes off the ground by rowing against the floor.

Note:
Keep your neck straight, and tighten your glutes and abs.

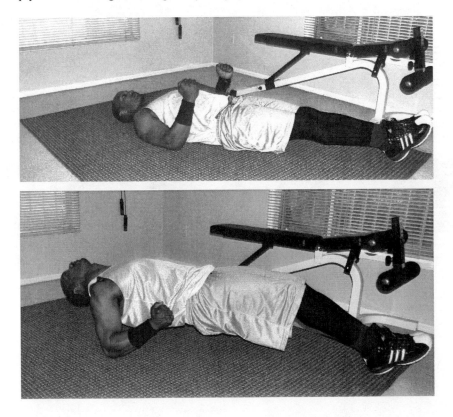

UPPER BODY PULLING EXERCISES

Elevated Horizontal Row

Beginning Position:
Use a ball, bench, or six-inch box. Lie on the floor with your back on the ground, knees bent, and feet flat on a ball, bench, or six-inch box.

Action:
Position your elbows eight inches away from your body and lift your shoulders, back, and glutes as high as you can.

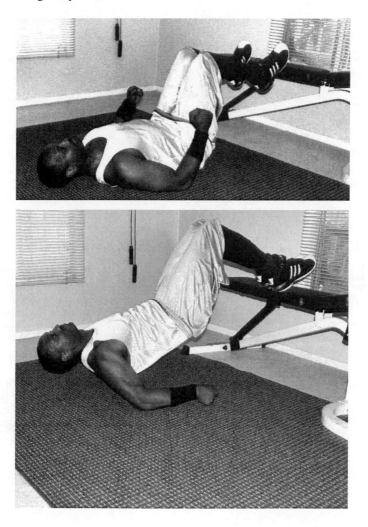

UPPER BODY PULLING EXERCISES

Single Arm Horizontal Row

Beginning Position:
Start by lying on your side with your knees bent and your elbow on the floor at approximately 30-45 degrees of lateral flexion in the shoulder.

Action:
Pull yourself up by pressing your elbow against the floor

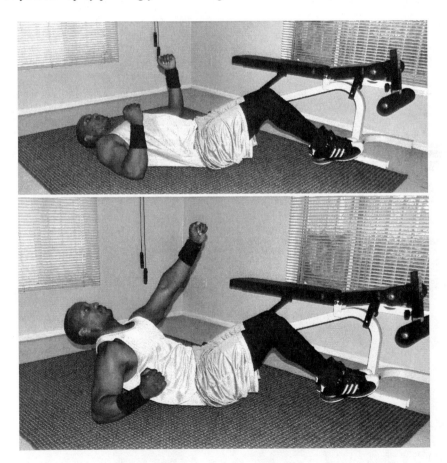

Upper Body Pushing Exercises

UPPER BODY PUSHING EXERCISES

Modified Push-up

Beginning Position:
Start while kneeling on the floor, place your arms slightly beyond shoulder width.

Action:
Push yourself up and lower yourself down.

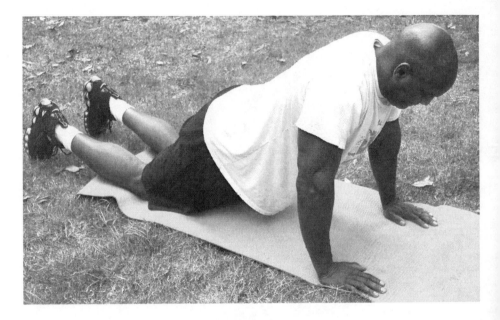

UPPER BODY PUSHING EXERCISES

Push-up

Beginning Position:
Start while lying on the floor with palms down, slightly shoulder-width apart.

Action:
While keeping your body straight, push against the floor until your arms are fully extended.

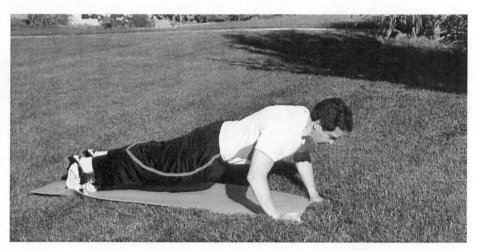

UPPER BODY PUSHING EXERCISES

Wide Push-up

Beginning Position:
Start by lying on the floor in the standard push-up position, place your hands six inches wider than your shoulder width.

Action:
Press against the floor until your arms are fully extended.

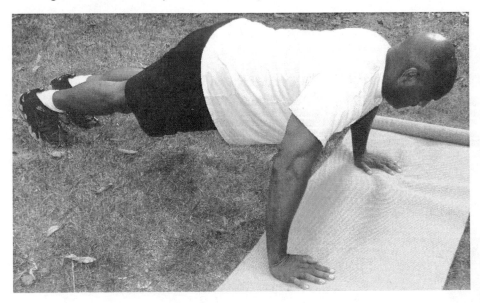

UPPER BODY PUSHING EXERCISES

Elevated Wide Push-up

Beginning Position:
Start with your feet on a box or on a bench and your chest on the floor, place your hands six inches wider than your shoulder width.

Action:
Press against the floor until your elbows are fully extended.

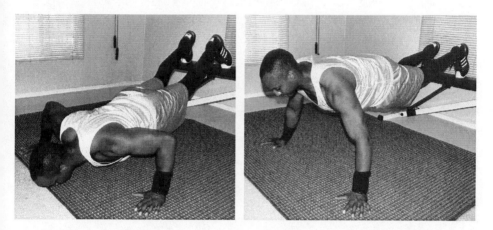

UPPER BODY PUSHING EXERCISES

Dive Bomber Push-up

Beginning Position:
Place yourself in the standard push-up position. Place your feet beyond shoulder-width apart and elevate your hips.

Action:
Lower your body using a diving motion. As your shoulders pass your wrist, extend and lock out your arms. Return by reversing the diving motion until your hips are elevated and in the starting position.

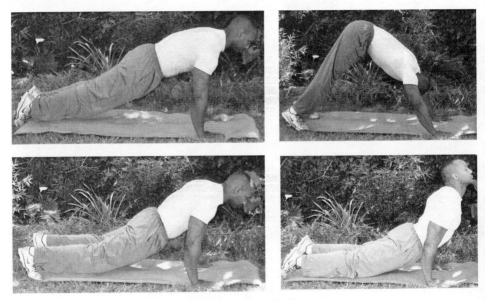

Photo by Aldonia Bailey

UPPER BODY PUSHING EXERCISES

Compression Push-up

Beginning Position:
Start while in the standard push-up position.

Action:
Place your feet flat against a wall. As you perform a push-up, push back and up to keep tension on your whole body.

Note:
Be sure to keep the entire soles of your feet on the wall.

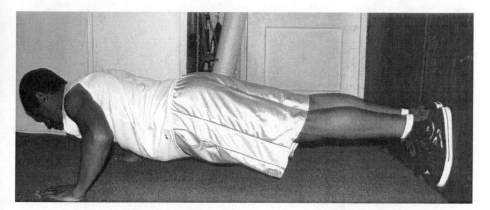

UPPER BODY PUSHING EXERCISES

Elevated Compression Push-up

Beginning Position:
While in the standard push-up position, place your feet six to twelve inches above the floor and flat against the wall.

Action:
As you perform a push-up, be sure to push back against the wall to keep tension on your entire body

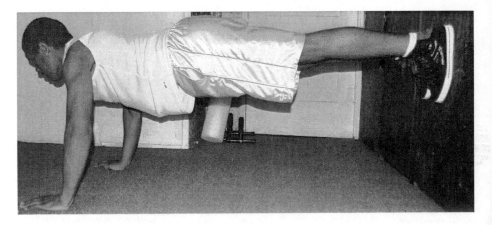

UPPER BODY PUSHING EXERCISES

Lateral Push-up/Side to Side

Beginning Position:
Start while in push-up position with your hands slightly wider than shoulder-width apart

Action:
Lower your body and place your body weight on one side. Return to the starting position and switch to the other side.

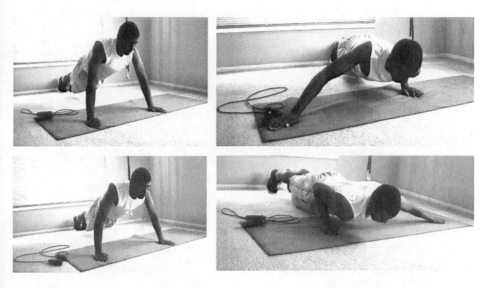

UPPER BODY PUSHING EXERCISES

Circle Push-up

Beginning Position:
Start while lying on the floor in the standard push-up position.

Action:
Lower one side of your body, and shift your body weight to the other side as you extend your arms, moving in a circular pattern.

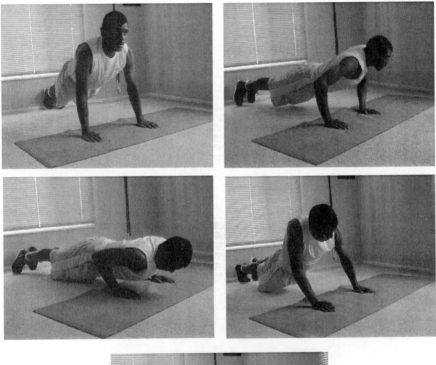

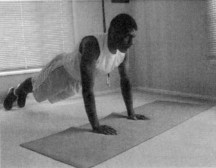

UPPER BODY PUSHING EXERCISES

Diamond Push-up

Beginning Position:
Start while lying on the floor with your feet shoulder-width apart, place your index fingers and thumbs together to form a diamond.

Action:
Push up against the floor until your arms are fully extended. Be careful not to flare your elbows away from your body.

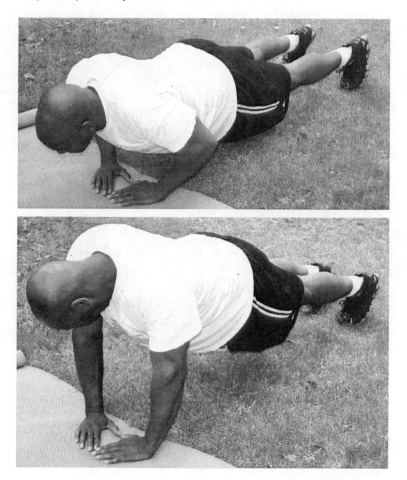

UPPER BODY PUSHING EXERCISES

Kneeling One-arm Push-up

Beginning Position:
Start with your knees on the floor, place one hand in the center of your body under your chest.

Action:
While keeping your arm close to your body, push yourself up.

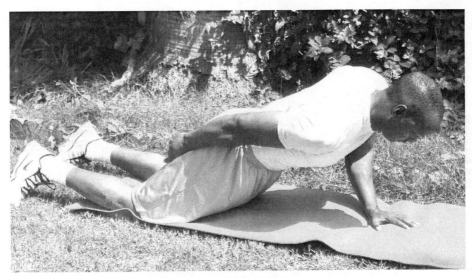

Photo by Aldonia Bailey

Modified One-arm Push-up

Beginning Position:
Start in push-up position, place your non-pushing arm on the floor or a ball.

Action:
Push yourself up with one arm.

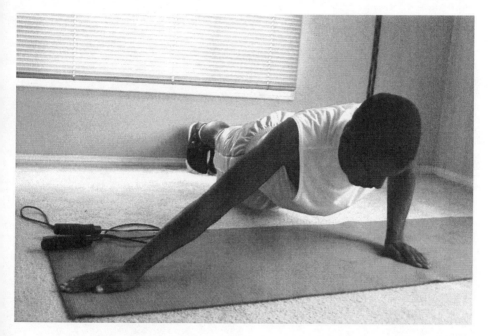

UPPER BODY PUSHING EXERCISES

One-arm Push-up

Beginning Position:
Start with your feet on the floor beyond shoulder-width apart and one hand in the center of your body under your chest.

Action:
While keeping your arm close to your body, push yourself up.

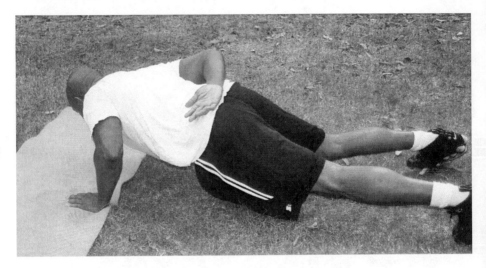

UPPER BODY PUSHING EXERCISES

Push-up Handle Side Push-up

Beginning Position:
Start by lying on your side with your body straight, place the push-up handle close to your body and in front of your chest.

Action:
Remain on your side and push yourself up.

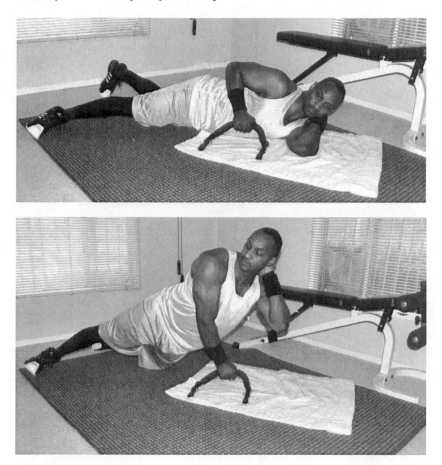

UPPER BODY PUSHING EXERCISES

Clapping Push-up

Beginning Position:
Start while you are lying on the floor in the standard push-up position.

Action:
Press against the floor with so much force that you can lift your hands and clap them. Make sure you land on your palms with your elbows bent.

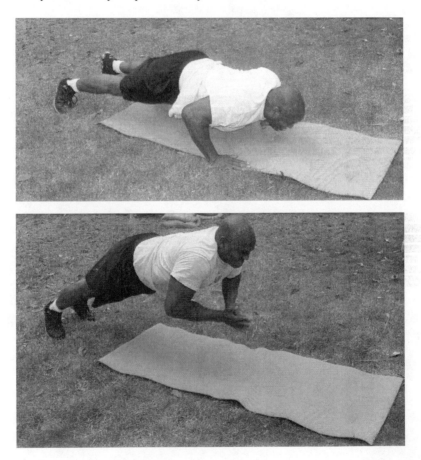

UPPER BODY PUSHING EXERCISES

Planche push up

Beginning Position:
Lying on the floor in the push up position. Place your hands close to you ab muscles
Keep your body straight and as stiff as possible

Action:
Push your whole body up and off of the floor.

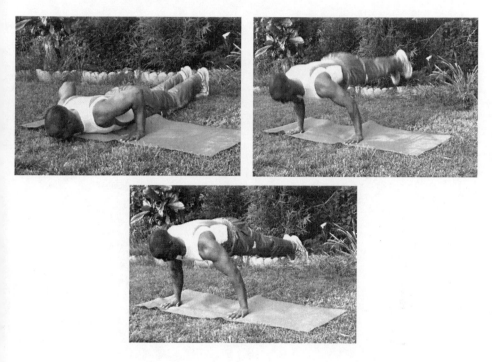

UPPER BODY PUSHING EXERCISES

Handstand

Beginning Position:
Place your hands shoulder-width apart.

Action:
Bend your knees as you thrust, and kick your legs up into a handstand.

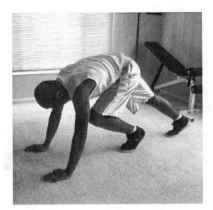

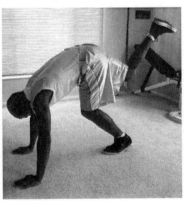

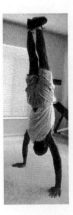

UPPER BODY PUSHING EXERCISES

Handstand Push-up

Beginning Position:
Start while in a handstand position and in front of a wall for add support.

Action:
Lower your body until your head is slightly off of the floor. Press yourself up to complete your rep.

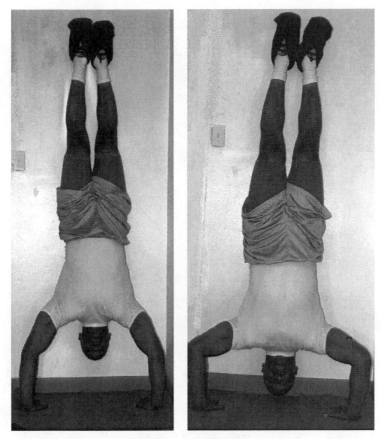

Photo by Aldonia Bailey

ADDITIONAL UPPER BODY PUSHING EXERCISES

UPPER BODY PUSHING EXERCISES

Lateral Wall Walking

Handstand Push-up

Beginning Position:
Start while in a handstand push-up position.

Action:
Bend your arms and walk along the wall. Every time you step with your hands, slide your feet against the wall. Straighten your arms after your right and left step is complete.

UPPER BODY PUSHING EXERCISES

One-Arm Handstand Push-up

Beginning Position:
Place your hands shoulder-width apart in front of a wall for added support.

Action:
Bend your knees as you thrust, and kick your legs up into a handstand. Lift one hand up and begin to lower yourself, and press yourself up with one arm.

Lower Body
Exercises

LOWER BODY EXERCISES

Step-Up

Beginning Position:
Start while standing with your front leg on a box or bench and flexed ninety degrees.

Action:
Use your front leg to stand on top of the box or bench.

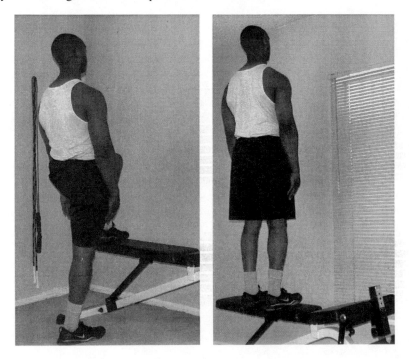

LOWER BODY EXERCISES

Wall Squat

Beginning Position:
Start with your back against the wall.

Action:
Lower your body as you walk away from the wall until your knees are flexed to ninety degrees. Your knees should also be in alignment with your feet, but not in front of your toes. Hold this position as you attempt to push against the wall.

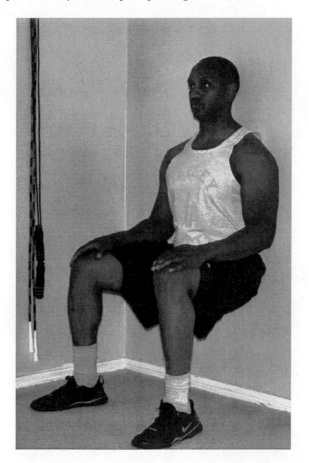

LOWER BODY EXERCISES

Single-leg Wall Squat

Beginning Position:
Start while standing with your feet shoulder-width apart and your body supported against a wall.

Action:
Squat down to lower your body until your knees are flexed at ninety degrees. Lift one leg off the ground and hold that position for a time. Repeat the exercise on both legs.

Note:
Keep your back flat against the wall.

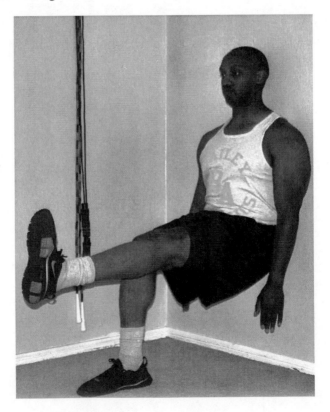

LOWER BODY EXERCISES

Squat

Beginning Position:
Stand straight up with your feet shoulder-width apart.

Action:
Bend your knees as you squat down. While keeping your back flat and chest up, continue to lower your body until you have reached 90 percent or lower. Make sure your knees are aligned over your feet. Stand up to repeat your set.

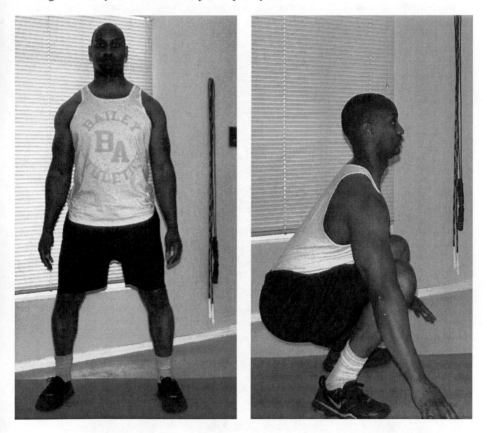

LOWER BODY EXERCISES

3-D Squat and Tap

Beginning Position:
Stand with your feet shoulder-width apart.

Action:
Squat down and tap the floor in the following sequence: Left hand touches by your left foot. Slightly stand up. Squat down again to touch the floor between both feet. Slightly stand up to touch the floor on the side of your right foot. Repeat the exercise with both hands.

Note:
Keep your chest up and your knees aligned over your feet.

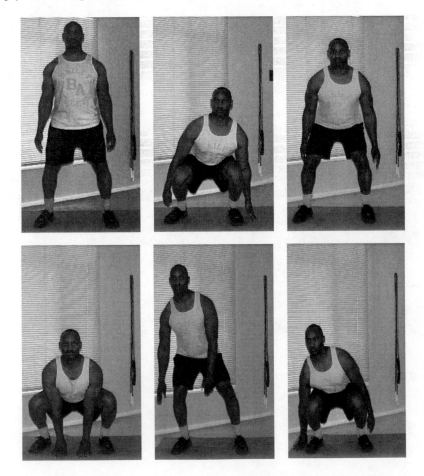

LOWER BODY EXERCISE

Deep Sumo Squat

Beginning Position:
Standing with your feet beyond shoulder width apart. Keep your knees in alignment with your toes as you slightly turn your feet out.

Action:
Mimic a Sumo Wrestler by squatting as low as you can. Stand up to complete your reps.

Return to your starting position & repeat the exercise

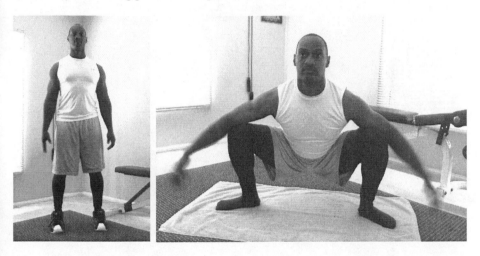

LOWER BODY EXERCISE

Sumo Squat Walk

Beginning Position:
Standing with your feet beyond shoulder with apart. Keep your knees in alignment with your toes as you slightly turn your feet out.

Action:
Mimic a Sumo Wrestler by squatting as low as you can and walk in the low sumo squat position complete your reps or walk for a predetermined distance.

Return to your starting position & repeat the exercise

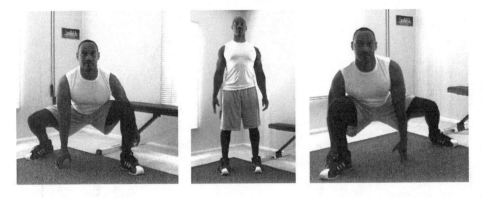

LOWER BODY EXERCISES

Lunge

Beginning Position:
Stand straight up with one leg in front of the other. With your feet placed with enough width to allow ninety degrees of flexion in your knees.

Action:
Keep your body weight on the front leg and your heel up on your back leg. Bend both knees and perform your reps.

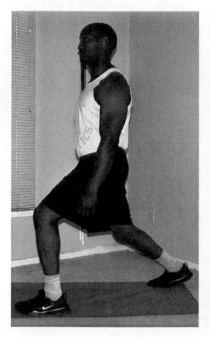
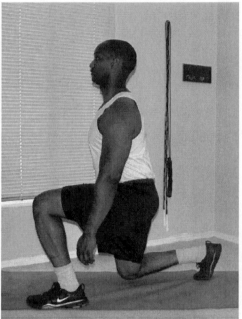

LOWER BODY EXERCISES

Acceleration/Deceleration Lunge

Beginning Position:
Start while standing with your feet hip-width apart.

Action:
Step forward with your lunging leg. When your lunging leg is off the floor, use your back leg to thrust and accelerate your body weight forward. When your front leg makes contact with the floor, immediately push with your front leg to thrust your body weight, and land with your lunging leg behind you with ninety degrees flexion in both knees. Repeat the movement on both legs.

Note: The back leg will accelerate the forward lunge and decelerate on the return. The front leg will decelerate upon landing of the front lunge and accelerate the return.

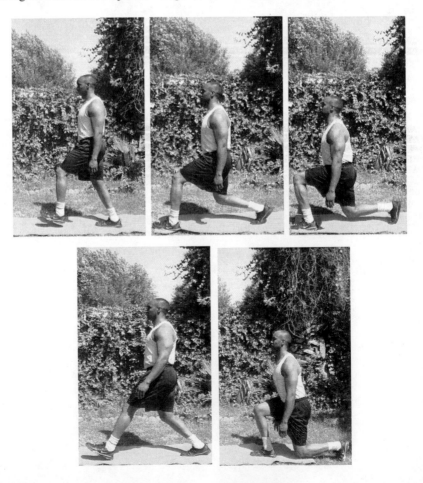

LOWER BODY EXERCISES

Duck Walks

Beginning Position:
Start while in a squat position with your heels in the air.

Action:
Walk while in the squatting position.

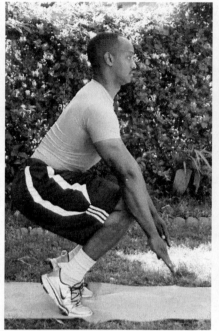 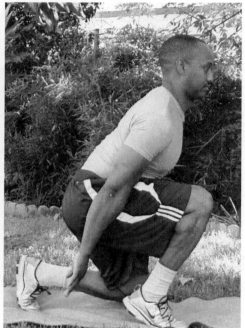

LOWER BODY EXERCISES

Transverse Duck Walk

Beginning Position:
Start while in the squat position, with your heels in the air.

Action:
Step to your left or right as you turn your knee and foot in the same direction. To complete the movement, step with your other leg and align your feet together. Alternate your legs as you cover your desired area.

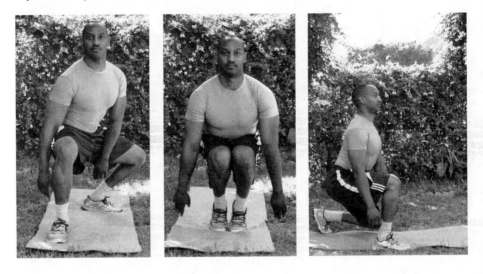

LOWER BODY EXERCISES

Lateral Lunge

Beginning Position:
Stand with your feet hip-width apart.

Action:
Use one leg to step out to your side and bend your leg. Keep the knee of your support leg directly over your big toe.

Note:
Go as low as you can without hunching over.

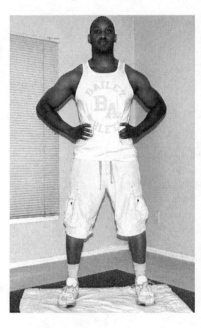 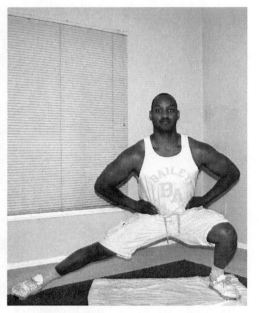

Lower Body Exercises

Crossover Lunge

Beginning Position:
Stand straight up with your feet shoulder-width apart. If possible, imagine yourself facing a clock. You are in the center of the clock, directly behind 12.

Action:
When using your right leg, step forward and over toward ten o'clock. Allow the heel of your hind leg to come up. Return to your starting position and step forward and over toward two o'clock with your left leg.

Note: Allow both knees to bend.

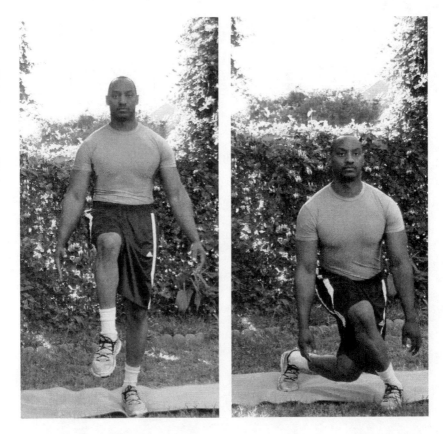

LOWER BODY EXERCISES

Woodchopper

Beginning Position:
Stand with your feet slightly beyond shoulder-width apart. Place your hands over your head with an air axe.

Action:
Bend your knees and perform a chopping movement.
As you chop downward, accelerate the movement by straightening your legs.

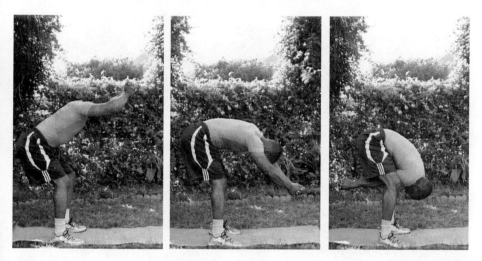

LOWER BODY EXERCISES

One-leg Supported Squat

Beginning Position:
Start while standing in a front lunge position, with your back leg supported by a step or bench and flexed ninety degrees at the knee.

Action:
Lower your body using your front leg. Use the same leg to push up to return to your starting position.

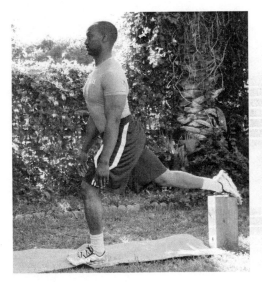 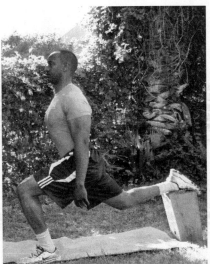

LOWER BODY EXERCISES

One-leg Supported Squat Jump

Beginning Position:
Start while standing in a front lunge position, with your back leg supported by a step or a bench and flexed ninety degrees at the knee.

Action:
Perform a one-leg squat and jump up. Be sure to keep your back leg on the bench when you are in the air.

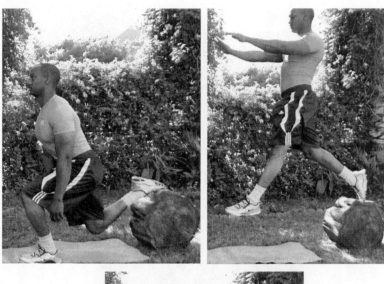

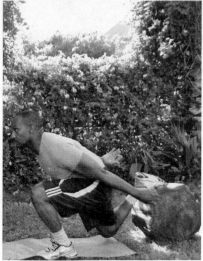

LOWER BODY EXERCISES

Ice Skater

Beginning Position:
Start while standing in the quarter squat position.

Action:
Jump laterally with one leg. Land on one foot, immediately push off, and jump laterally in the opposite direction.

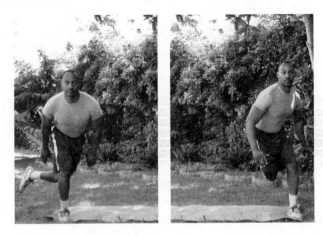

LOWER BODY EXERCISE

Box jump

Beginning Position:
While standing in front of a plyo-box or bench.

Action:
Jump up & land on the box.

Return to your starting position & repeat the exercise.

LOWER BODY EXERCISES

Jumping Jack Squat

Beginning Position:
Start while in a squat position with your arms to your side.

Action:
Jump up and out of the squat to perform your jumping jack.

Return to your starting position and repeat the exercise.

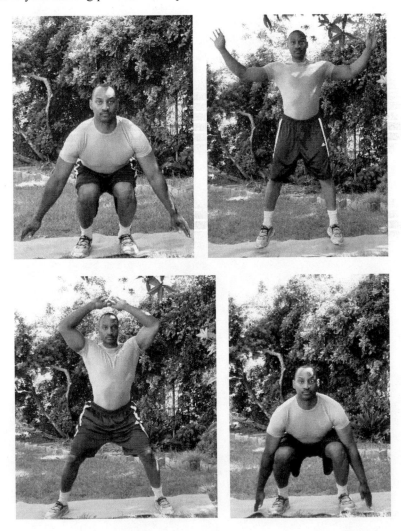

LOWER BODY EXERCISES

Frog Jump

Beginning Position:
Start while in a deep squat position, with your hands touching the floor and arms bent with shoulders elevated.

Action:
Mimic a frog by jumping or hopping up using your legs. Assist your movement by simultaneously depressing your shoulders and pushing off the ground with your hands.

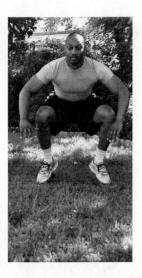

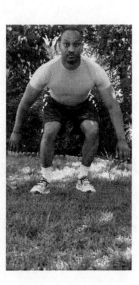

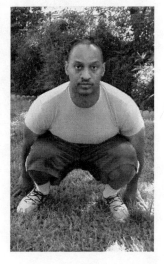

LOWER BODY EXERCISES

Lateral Frog Jump

Beginning Position:
Start while in a deep squat position, with your hands touching the floor, arm bent, and shoulders elevated.

Action:
Mimic a frog by jumping or hopping to your left or right side. Assist your jumping movement by simultaneously depressing your shoulders and pushing off the ground with your hands.

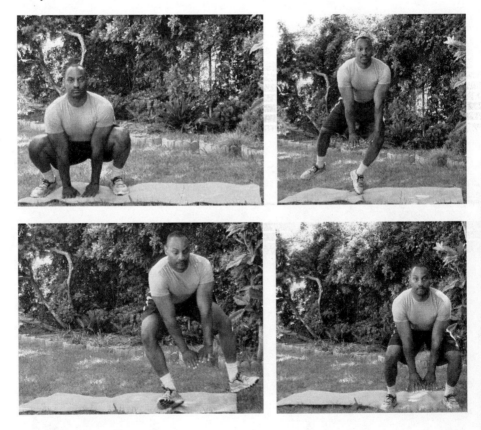

Split Jump Lunge

Beginning Position:
Start while standing in the lunge position.

Action:
Jump up from the lunge position, and in the lunge position, repeat the exercise using the same leg.

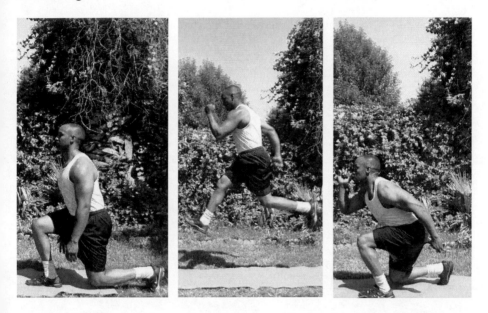

LOWER BODY EXERCISES

Modified Kick-outs

Beginning Position:
Start while standing in a deep squat position.

Action:
Bounce up to the standing ninety-degree squat position and kick your leg out.

Repeat by returning to the starting position and alternating to your other leg.

To increase the intensity, do not alternate between squats for all of your reps on one leg. To complete the set, perform the same amount of reps on your other leg.

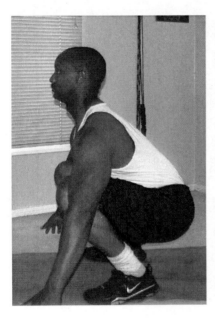
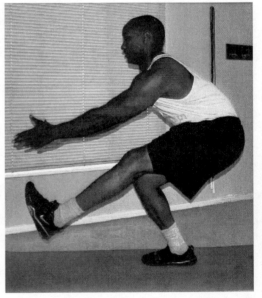

LOWER BODY EXERCISES

Single-leg Squat

Beginning Position:
Stand with your feet hip-width apart, squat down ninety degrees.

Action:
Lift one leg off the ground and stand up on one leg. Be sure to stand up and lower yourself with one leg to count the rep.

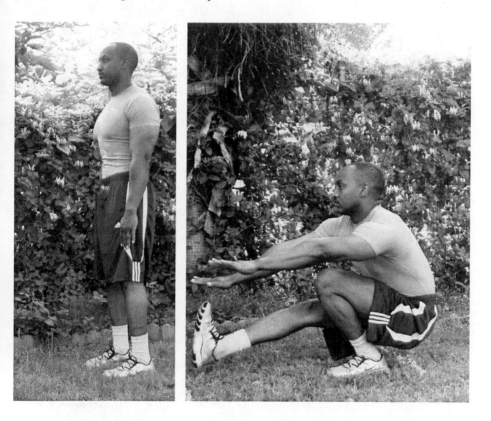

LOWER BODY EXERCISE

BA—Wave squat

This version of the wave squat is taken from Bailey Athletics.
Beginning position: Stand in the standard squatting position.

Action:
1 repetition BA—wave squat is equal to 4 reps of a regular squat.
Perform the squats without stopping or pausing. 2 quarter squats—1 full squat jump—1
squat jump. Be sure to land with your knees bent.

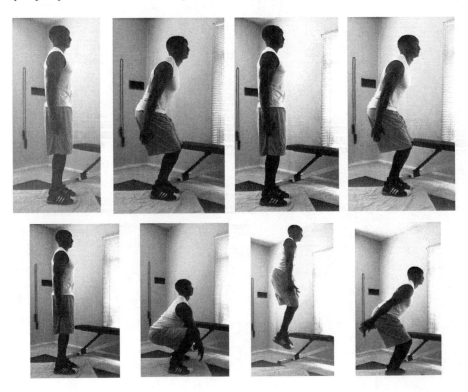

LOWER BODY EXERCISES

Broad Jump

Beginning Position:
Start while standing with your feet shoulder-width apart, with a slight bend in your knees and hips.

Action:
Explosively jump forward using your legs and arms. Land with your chest up with bent knees

Note:
Jump as far as you can.

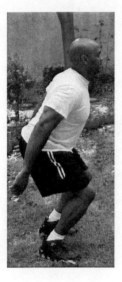
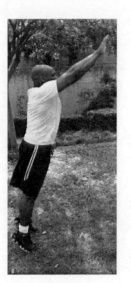
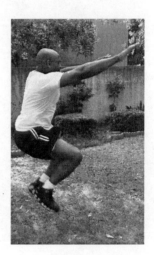

LOWER BODY EXERCISES

Tuck Jump

Beginning Position:
Start while standing with your feet shoulder-width apart.

Action:
Squat down and jump up.
While in the air, pull your knees to your chest and let go before you land.

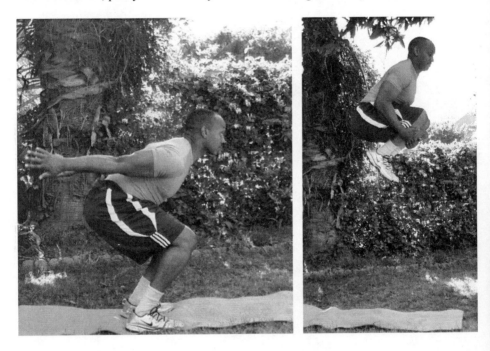

Transverse Jump Squat

Beginning Position:
Stand straight up with your feet shoulder-width apart.

Action:
Bend your knees and jump. While in the air, rotate your body to your left or right. Upon landing, immediately perform the same movement to your opposite side.

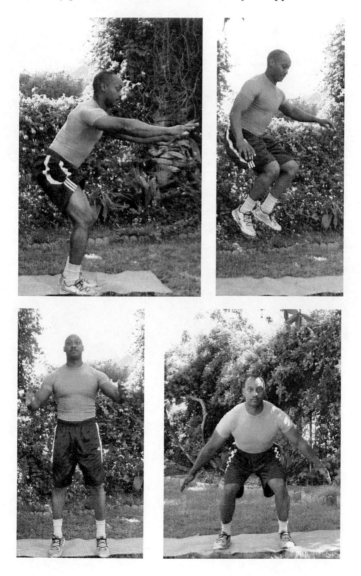

ABDOMINAL EXERCISES

Core

Body Rolling

Beginning Position:
Start while lying on your back with your legs slightly elevated. Place your arms straight and over your head.

Action:
Lift your chest, arm, and legs to roll your body completely over. Be sure to elevate your chest when you are on your stomach or your back.

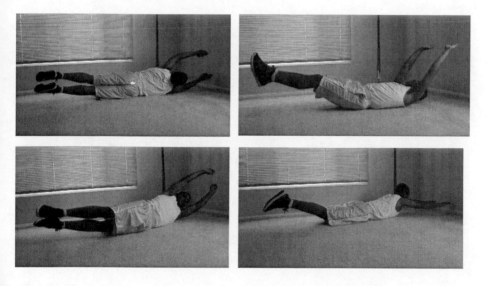

ABDOMINAL EXERCISES
Core

Planks

Beginning Position:
Start with your chest facing down on the floor.

Action:
Hold your body up off of the floor by resting on your forearms, elbows, and toes. Keep your back and head straight as you contract your abs by tucking your hips inward toward your arms.

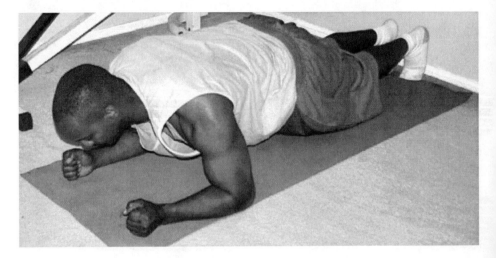

ABDOMINAL EXERCISES
Core

Single-leg Planks

Beginning Position:
Lie on the floor by holding your body up by resting on your forearms, elbows, and toes.

Action:
Lift your right or left leg in the air. Keep your back and head straight as you contract your abs by tucking your hips inward toward your arms. Perform this exercise on both legs.

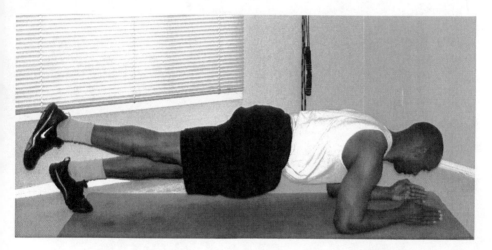

ABDOMINAL EXERCISES
Core

Single-leg Elevated Plank

Beginning Position:
Start while in the plank position. Place one leg on a bench.

Action:
Lift and support your body on the bench. Keep your other leg straight and in the air, off the bench. Hold the position for time or perform reps.

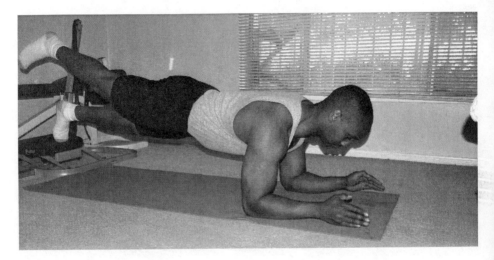

Abdominal Exercises
Core

Side Plank

Beginning Position:
Start on your side with your hips in the air.

Action:
Support and balance yourself on one forearm and the side of your foot.

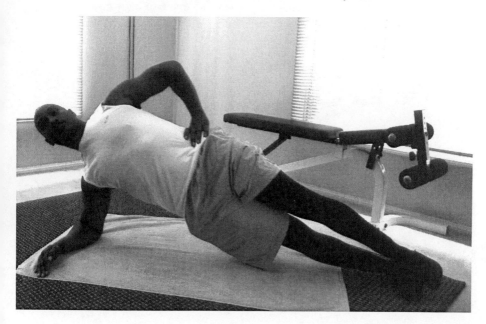

ABDOMINAL EXERCISES
Core

Elevated Leg Side Plank

Beginning Position:
Start on your side with your hips in the air.

Action:
Support and balance yourself on on your one arm and one foot. Elevate and lift the leg that is not touching the floor.

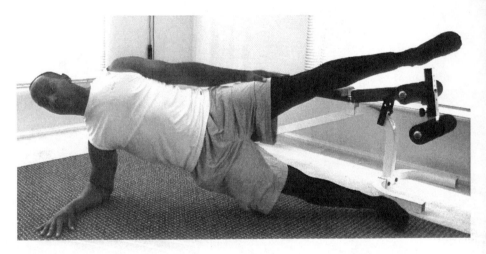

ABDOMINAL EXERCISES
Core

Elevated Single-leg Side Plank

Beginning Position:
Lie on your side with your hips in the air.

Action:
Support and balance your body with your bottom foot supported on a bench and your top leg straight in the air. Hold the position for a time or perform reps.

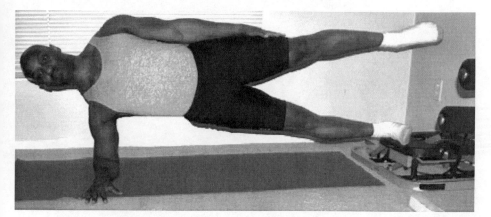

ABDOMINAL EXERCISES
Core

Medial Side Plank

Beginning Position:
Start while in a side plank position. Place your top leg on the floor.

Action:
Lift your body up. Place your bottom leg up in the air and slightly forward. Hold the position for a time or perform reps.

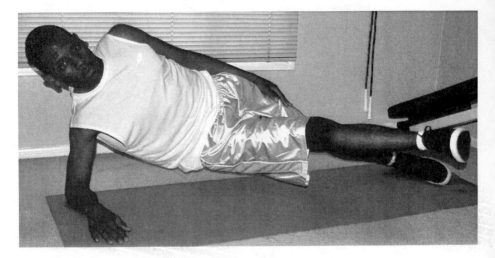

ABDOMINAL EXERCISES
Core

Elevated Medial Side Plank

Beginning Position:
Start while in a side plank position,

Action:
Place your top leg on a bench and lift your body up. Place your bottom leg in the air and under the bench. Hold the position for a time or perform reps.

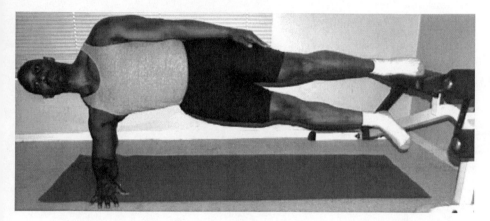

ABDOMINAL EXERCISES
Core

Elbow Bridge

Beginning Position:
While lying on your back, support your body on your elbows. Keep your legs straight and close together.

Action:
Lift your hips upward off the floor. Hold this position for a time or perform reps.

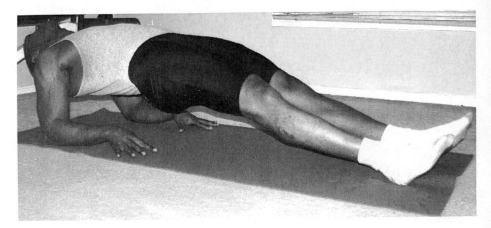

Abdominal Exercises
Core

Single-leg Elbow Bridge

Beginning Position:
Lie on your back and support your body on your elbows. Keep your legs straight and close together.

Action:
Lift your hips and one leg upward off the floor. Hold this position for a time or perform reps.

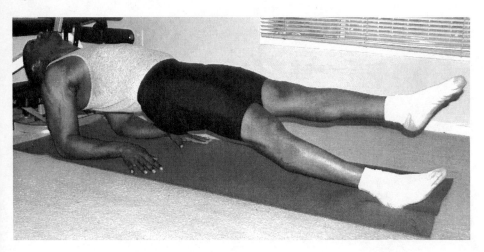

ABDOMINAL EXERCISES
Core

Elevated Single-leg Elbow Bridge

Beginning Position:
Lie on your back and support your body on your elbows. Place your feet on a bench with your legs straight and close together.

Action:
After you lift your hips upward off the floor, lift one leg off the bench. Hold this position for a time or perform reps.

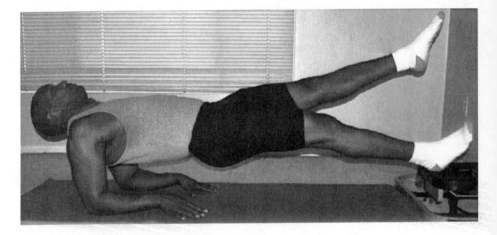

ABDOMINAL EXERCISES
Core

Elevated Single-leg Hip Extension

Beginning Position:
Lie on your back and support your body on your elbows.

Action:
Place and bend one leg or foot on a bench and lift your body upward. Keep your back and hips straight as you hold the position for a time or perform reps.

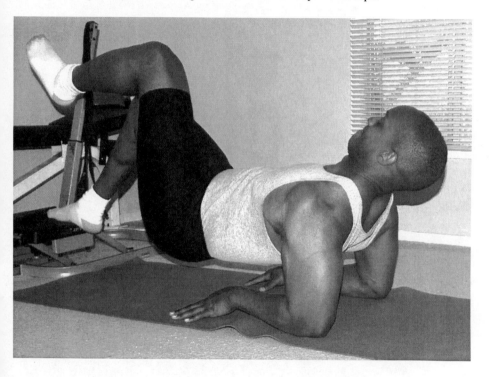

ABDOMINAL EXERCISES
Upper/Lower/Obliques

Rocking Bicycle Crunch

Beginning Position
Start while lying on the floor with your fingers locked behind your neck and knees bent.

Action:
Rock your body backward and forward. As you allow yourself to rock, extend your legs to mimic the cycling motion while simultaneously rotating your waist and shoulders to touch your knees with your elbows.

Try to touch the side of your leg with the side of your elbow.

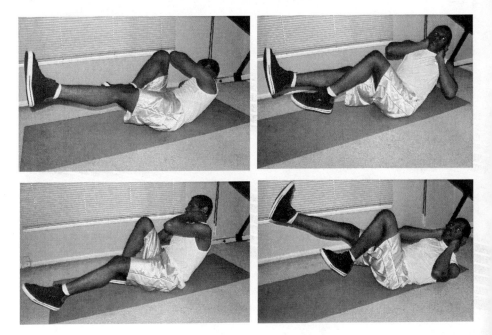

ABDOMINAL EXERCISES
Upper/Lower/Obliques

Stride Crunch

Beginning Position:
Start on your back while lying on the floor with your legs bent at thirty degrees. Place your hands on your ear, your elbows in the air, and your chin on your chest.

Action:
Lift your leg up toward your elbows as if you are taking a long step/stride. Lift your back up and rotate your shoulders to bring your opposite elbow to your leg. Return your leg to the floor and repeat the exercise on your other side.

Note:
Try to touch the opposite side of your leg with your elbow.

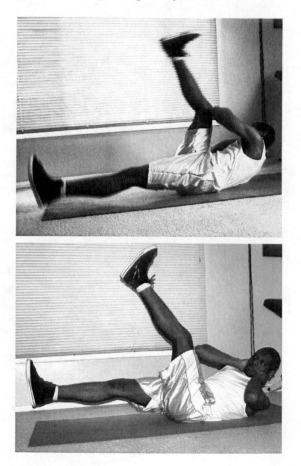

ABDOMINAL EXERCISES
Upper/Lower/Obliques

Bicycle Crunches

Beginning Position:
Lie on your back with your arms bent and hands by your ears.

Action:
Lift your leg as you bring your knee to touch your opposite elbow. Return your leg to the air and repeat the movement with your other side.

Notes:
1. Tuck your chin to your chest.
2. Try to touch the opposite side of your leg with your elbow.

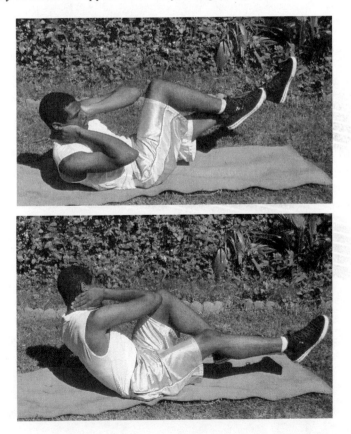

ABDOMINAL EXERCISES
Upper/Lower/Obliques

Hanging Circumduction

Beginning Position:
While hanging on a bar or pull up bar, raise your legs until your feet are above or at your shoulders.

Action:
Lower your legs toward your side. Make a circle with your legs by raising your legs to your other side.

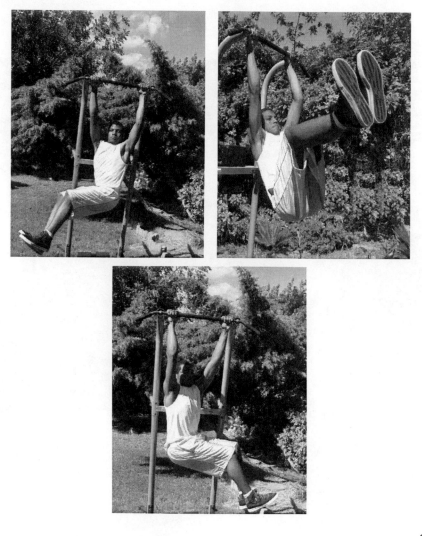

ABDOMINAL EXERCISES
Upper and Lower

Rocking Crunch

Beginning Position:
Lie on your back with your knees tucked to your chest. Place your chin on your chest. Place your hands behind your head and place your elbows on your knees.

Action:
Keep your elbows on your knees as you rock backward and forward without pausing.

Option: Place a sandbag between your elbows and your knees. Squeeze it as you rock.

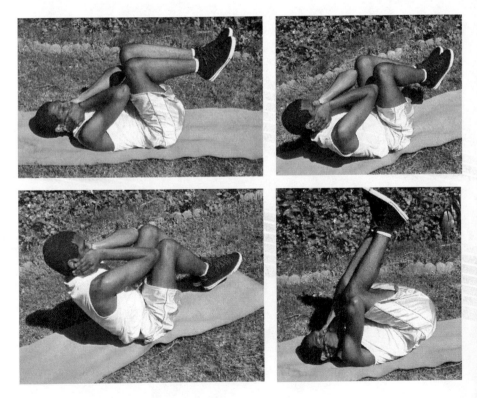

ABDOMINAL EXERCISES
Upper and Lower

Weighted Rocking Sit-up

Beginning Position:
Start by lying on your back with straight legs and your feet in the air, hold the sandbag over your head on your forearms.

Action:
Lift and pull the sandbag over your head as you tuck your knees in to meet your elbows. Sit up and rock forward. After your knees and elbows meet, rock backward to return to your starting position.

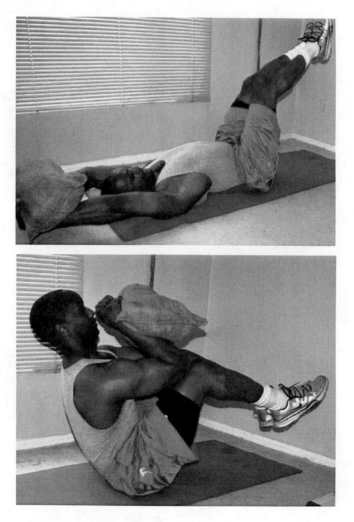

ABDOMINAL EXERCISES
Upper and Lower

Jackknife

Beginning Position:
Start while lying on your back with your legs straight and your arms stretched and straight over your head.

Action:
Simultaneously lift your arms and chest as you raise your legs to meet your chest to mimic a jackknife.

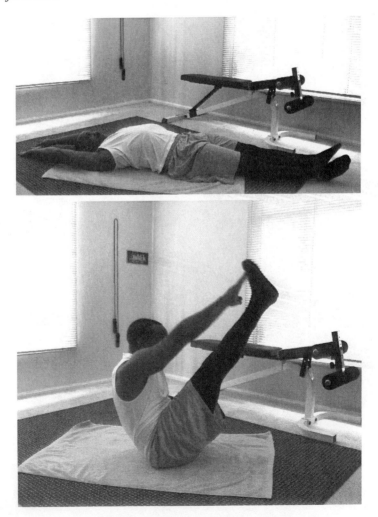

ABDOMINAL EXERCISES
Upper and Lower

Single-leg Jackknife

Beginning Position:
Start while lying on your back with your legs straight and your arms stretched and straight over your head.

Action:
Simultaneously lift your arms and chest to meet your legs. When your legs and chest are facing each other, touch your leg and repeat the exercise with your other leg.

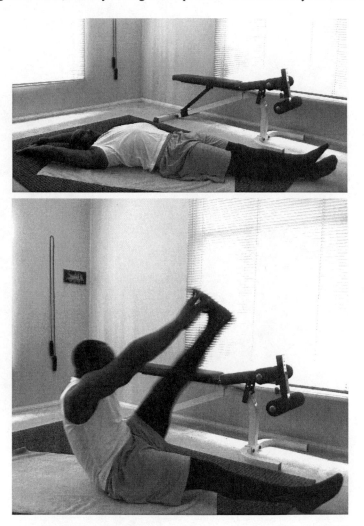

Lower

Lying Hip Lifts

Beginning Position:
Start while lying on your back with your arms at your side and your palms down.

Action:
Lift your legs until your hips are flexed to ninety degrees. Raise your hips up and off the floor. Try not to roll backward or move laterally. Lower your hips to the ground and repeat the movement for reps.

Note:
When lowering your legs, be careful not to arch your back.

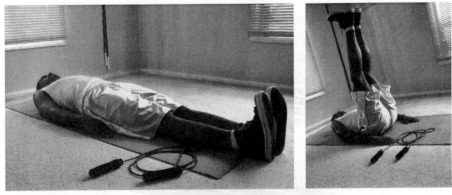

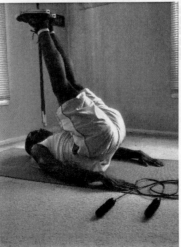

ABDOMINAL EXERCISES
Lower

Seated Leg Lifts

Beginning Position:
While sitting with your legs straight and your back upright, place your hands on the floor and lock your elbows.

Action:
Look straight ahead as you tuck your hips in, and gently lift your legs as high as you can or until your toes pass your chest with good form.

Notes:
1. Hand placements vary due to arm length. Place your hands in a position that will allow you to keep your hips tucked in and hold your back upright.
2. When lowering your leg, be careful not to arch your back.

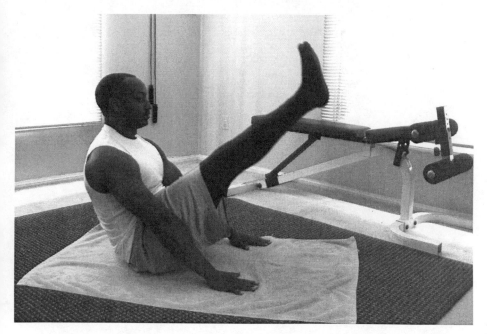

ABDOMINAL EXERCISES
Lower

Seated Single-leg Lifts

Beginning Position:
Start while sitting with your legs straight and your back upright.

Action:
Place your hands on the floor and lock your elbows. Look straight ahead as you tuck your hips in and lift your right or left leg as high as you can or until your toes pass your chest with good form.

Notes:
1. Hand placements vary due to arm length. Place your hands in a position that will allow you to keep your hips tucked in and hold your back upright.
2. When lowering your legs, be careful not to arch your back.

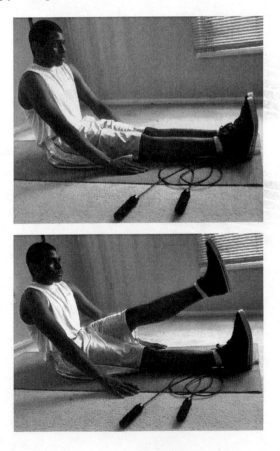

ABDOMINAL EXERCISES
Lower

Hanging Bent-knee Leg Lifts

Beginning Position:
Hang on a pull-up bar or straight bar.

Action:
Bend and raise your knees four-six inches above your navel.

Note:
When lowering your legs, be careful not to arch your back.

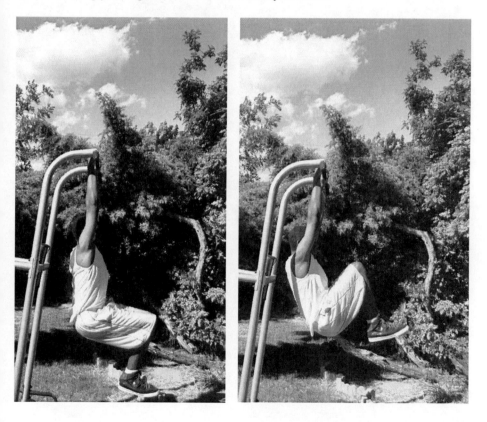

ABDOMINAL EXERCISES
Lower

Hanging Straight Leg Lifts

Beginning Position:
Start while hanging on a pull-up bar or a straight bar.

Action:
Raise your legs more than four inches above your navel.

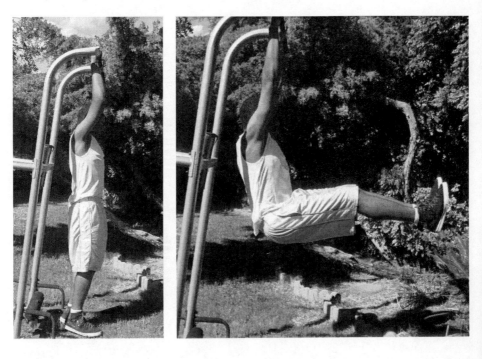

Note:
When lowering your legs, be careful not to arch your back.

Abdominal Exercises
Lower

Hanging Single-leg Lift

Beginning Position:
Start while hanging on a pull-up bar or a straight bar.

Action:
Raise your right or left leg more than four inches above your navel. Lower your leg and repeat the movement with your other leg.

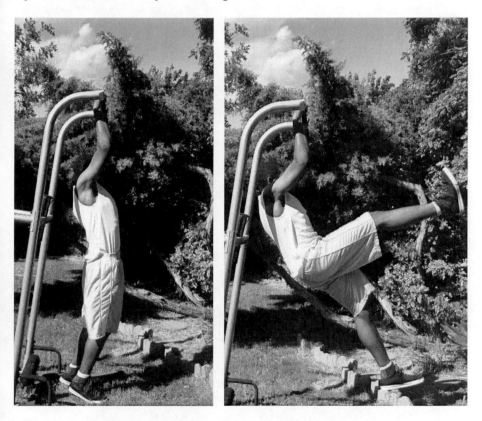

Note:
When lowering your legs, be careful not to arch your back.

ABDOMINAL EXERCISES
Obliques

Full-body Side Raise

Beginning Position:
Start while on your side with your bottom arm straight on the floor and your top arm at your side.

Action:
Simultaneously lift your chest, shoulders, and legs off the floor. Gently lower your chest, shoulders, and legs off the floor to reset your body to perform more reps.

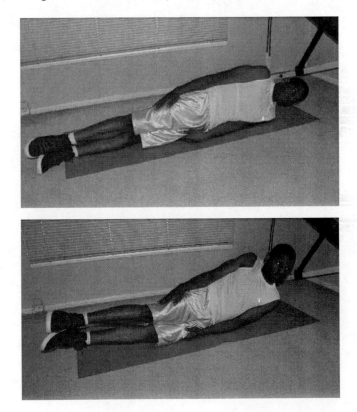

ABDOMINAL EXERCISES
Obliques

Seesaw Planks

Beginning Position:
Start while in the plank position.

Action:
Tap the floor using the side of your hip. After you touch the floor with your hip, return to the plank position and touch the floor with the other side of your hip.

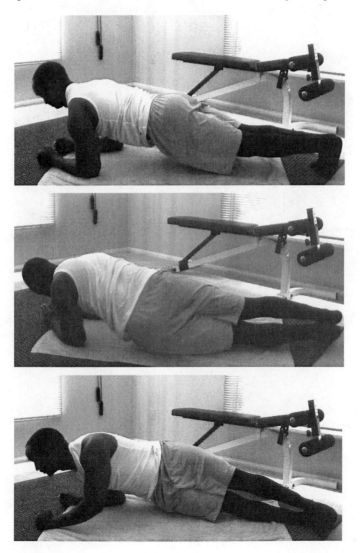

ABDOMINAL EXERCISES
Obliques

Windshield Wiper

Beginning Position:
Start while lying on your back with your arms 30-45 degrees away from your body.

Action:
Lift your legs up until your feet point toward the ceiling or sky. When your hips are at a ninety-degree flexion, gently lower your legs from one side to the other to mimic a windshield wiper.

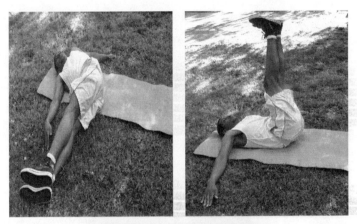

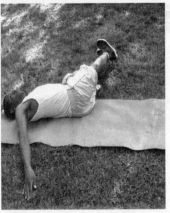

Abdominal Exercises
Upper

Crunches

Beginning Position:
Start while lying on your back with your knees bent.

Action:
Place your hands on your ears and touch your chin down toward your chest. Curl your chest and shoulders up toward your knees.

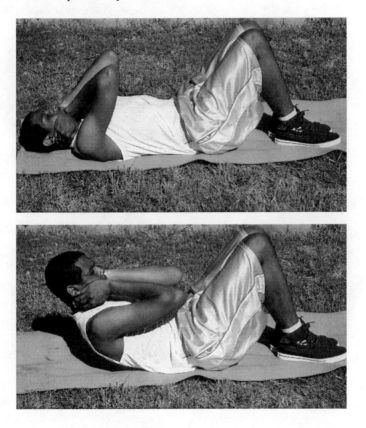

ABDOMINAL EXERCISES
Upper

Supported Jackknife

Beginning Position:
Start while lying on your back with your legs supported by a medicine ball or against a wall. Place your straight stretch arms straight over your head.

Action:
Simultaneously lift your arm and chest up off the floor toward your supported feet.

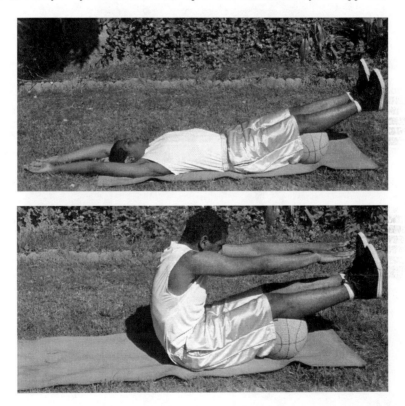

Abdominal Region
Back

Superman

Beginning Position:
Lie on your stomach with your legs straight and your arms straight over your head.

Action:
Raise your chest with your arms and legs straight in the air and return them to the floor. Repeat for a time or reps.

Note:
Contract your abdominals and glutes.

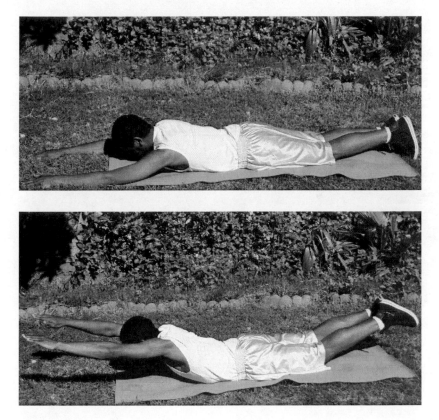

ABDOMINAL REGION
Back

Bridge

Beginning Position:
Start while lying on the floor with your knees bent and feet flat on the floor. Keep your body stable and tight.

Action:
Raise your hips and lower back off the floor until your hips are extended to zero degrees.

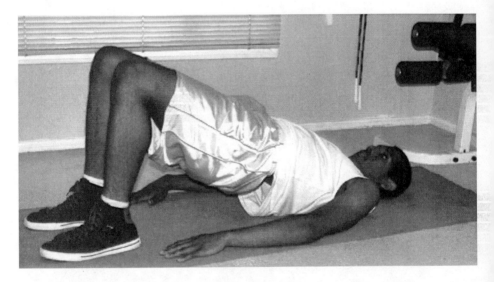

Note:
Keep your arms on the floor for more stability or on your chest for less stability.

ABDOMINAL REGION
Back

Single-leg Bridge

Beginning Position:
Start while lying on the floor with your knees bent and your feet flat on the floor. Keep your body stable and tight.

Action:
Raise one leg in the air and lift your hips and lower back off the floor until your hips are extended to zero degrees.

Note:
Keep your arms on the floor for more stability or on your chest for less stability

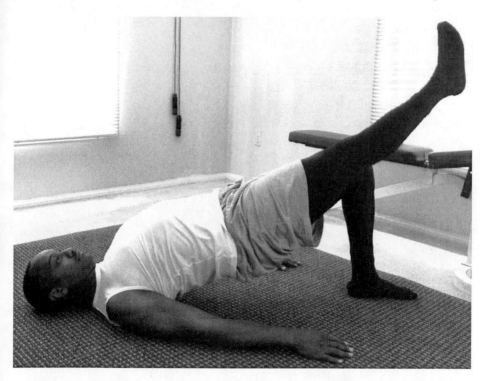

ABDOMINAL REGION
Back

Modified Full-body Bridge

Beginning Position:
Sit on a bench or a box that stands as high as your knees. Lie across the bench until only your shoulders are on the bench. Keep your knees and feet together with feet flat on the floor.

Action
Position your arms on the bench so that you're hands are facing your knees and your elbows are pointing at the sky. Stabilize your body as you use your hands, arms, shoulder, and hips to bridge.

Note: Try to push through your heels and squeeze your glutes at the peak of your contraction. Keep your knees together.

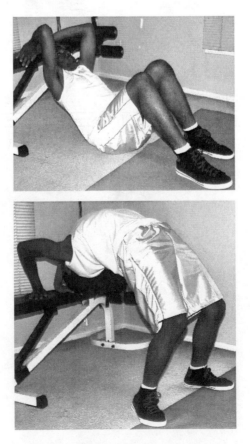

ABDOMINAL REGION
Back

Full-body Bridge

Beginning Position:
Start while lying on your back with your knees up and feet flat. Position your arms so that your hands and fingers are facing your knees and your elbows are pointing toward the sky.

Action:
Use your hands, arms, shoulders, and hips to elevate your body and bridge.

Note:
Keep your knees together.

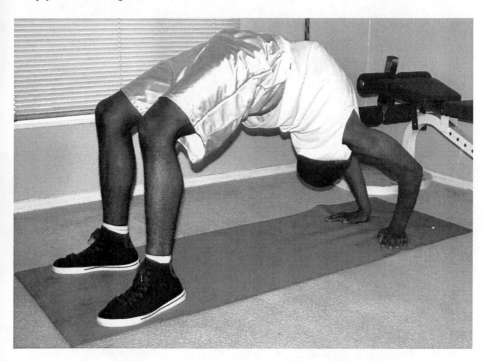

ABDOMINAL REGION
Back

Modified Single-leg Full-body Bridge

Beginning Position:
Position your body to perform a modified full-body bridge.

Action:
When you are in the full-body bridging position, perform the movement and lift one foot off the floor. Stabilize your body by squeezing and contracting your abs and glutes. Keep your knees and hips aligned. Do not allow your body to shift or move around. Perform this exercise on both legs.

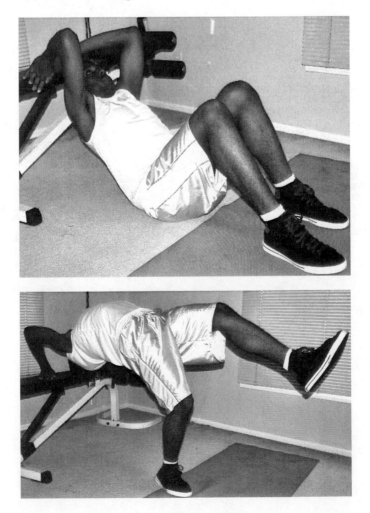

ABDOMINAL REGION
Back

Single-leg Full-body Bridge

Beginning Position:
Position your body to perform a full-body bridge. Lie on your back with your knees up and feet flat on the floor. Position your arms to be in the full bridge.

Action:
Perform a bridge and lift one foot off the floor. Keep your knees and hips aligned. Do not allow your body to shift or move around. Perform this exercise on both legs.

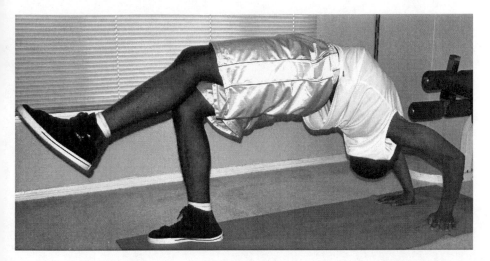

Chapter 3

Jump Rope Training

Jumping Rope

For years, people have used jump ropes to get in shape or to increase their levels of health and sport fitness. As a conditioning tool, many sports teams, fitness enthusiast, and professional athletes rely on jumping rope to contribute to their daily dose of aerobic and anaerobic conditioning.

Sports teams, fitness enthusiast, and professional athletes also rely on jumping rope to

- Supply an upper and lower body workout;
- tone muscle and burn fat;
- enhance coordination, speed, timing, rhythm, agility, and quickness;
- promote strong joints and ligaments; and
- increase aerobic and anaerobic conditioning

Tone Muscles and Burns Fat

Jumping rope requires that you use all of your upper and lower major muscle groups. Studies show that a low-level fifteen-minute jump rope routine provides an average size adult a caloric loss of about 150-200 calories (Solis:1992, 19). If you implement any tricky moves, you can burn more calories, allowing you to burn off up to a 1,000 calories in one hour!

Since one pound of fat is equal to 3,500 calories, if you burn off 1,000 calories in one hour, losing one pound of fat could take less than a week. Everybody wants to burn fat quickly, so, before you get started, do not forget the safety guidelines listed under the Safe topic.

ENHANCES COORDINATION, SPEED, TIMING, RHYTHM, AGILITY, AND QUICKNESS

The human body is so wonderfully designed that it can perform feats of physical task while mentally computing the exact amount of blood, hormones, and oxygen without any conscious thought. Jumping rope is a great testimony to this fact and can be explained by something known as chronic adaptation. Chronic adaptation is responsible for the phrase "perfect practice makes perfect." The phrase holds true because our bodies will learn what we teach it.

Enhanced muscle coordination, speed, timing, rhythm, agility, and quickness are required to jump rope efficiently. Through chronic adaptation or, put simply, long-term practice of short and long sessions of well-performed jump rope routines will result in positive changes to your central nervous system, muscle skeletal system, and body control (e.g., muscle coordination, speed, timing, rhythm, agility, and quickness).

Jumping rope involves a certain cadence per task and, therefore, is just as good as running through tires, cones, and ladders to attain the enhanced movement that you desire.(Solis; 1992:25)

PROMOTES STRONG BONES JOINTS AND LIGAMENTS

Our world is gravity based. Everything on the planet is compressed against gravity. As we age and become gradually weaker, gravity does not; it stays strong. If we are not making progress, then we are going backwards, getting weaker. Every day, our bodies require physical exertion to release vitamins like calcium to stay strong and adapt to our atmosphere. Without the right kind of physical activity, like low-level impact exercises, our bones, joints, and ligaments will not have the need to adapt. For those who are almost over the "non-active living" fence, I sometimes have to ask the hard questions, like, if you're not going to adapt to your atmosphere (e.g., gravity), then how do you expect your body to respond when you need it most?

SAFE

Jumping rope *is made* safe by taking precautions like selecting the type of floor you work out on. Wood, rubber, and any other kind of shock-absorbing floor that rebounds will decrease the impact on your body. Jump rope in an area that is at least nine and a half feet in diameter and in height to avoid things around you. Studies from many published researchers have shown that jumping rope is an excellent exercise, and it is also important to use the proper jump rope technique to avoid injury and make progress.

Jumping slower than what most suggest as the average amount of rotations, 120 rpm-130 rpm requires jumping higher or pausing between jumps to maintain the timing for a successful rope rotation.

If you are new to jumping rope, you want to take note that selecting the right length jump rope is the first step to not whipping yourself. The majority of your discomfort while jumping rope should come from fatigue. It's good to be tough, but it's better to be tough, healthy, and injury free.

Pausing when fatigued and using the matador open jump rope exercise (listed in the Jump Rope Exercise section) to catch your breath will give your body time to recover and complete your routine without getting injured. This technique resembles interval training because you are *interchanging short periods of jumping with non-jumping skills*, which decreases your aerobic demands and, again, dramatically reduces the chances of getting an overuse injury.

EASY TO LEARN

A great way to start your jump rope routine is to perform the movements of the exercise without having the jump rope in your hand. This is called a movement-specific training and is also a great way to warm up. This movement-specific warm-up is especially helpful for learning new jump rope skills. For your convenience, I've listed a few tips to help you safely learn to jump rope with ease.

GOT THE RIGHT JUMP ROPE?

1. Your rope should turn easily within the handles with or without bearings.
2. The right length jump rope for you will allow the part of the handle that touches the rope to meet (not pass) your armpits while you are standing on the jump rope with one or both feet.
3. Use a rope that feels right to your hand size.
4. Use wrist bands or jump ropes with foam on the handles if you're prone to heavy sweating and or sweaty palms.
5. Segmented ropes are great for overall jump roping.
6. Cotton ropes or soft ropes rotate slower than other jump ropes. It's mainly used to learn new techniques.
7. Weighted ropes are recommended for people with good muscle-skeletal conditioning.

Jump Rope Training References

(1) Ken M. Solis; Ropics, 1992:19
(2) (Ken M. Solis; Ropics, 1992:25

Chapter 4

Jump Rope Exercises

JUMP ROPE EXERCISES

Figure Eight

Beginning Position:
Stand in a stationary position.

Action:
Turn the rope from one side to the other (left to right and right to left) as you outline a figure eight in the air.

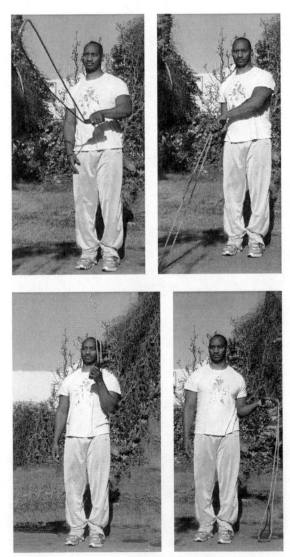

Matador Open

Beginning Position:
Swing the rope with both hands from one side to the other side.

Action:
Open and widen your arms to allow the rope to pass over you as you jump through the rope after each side rotation.

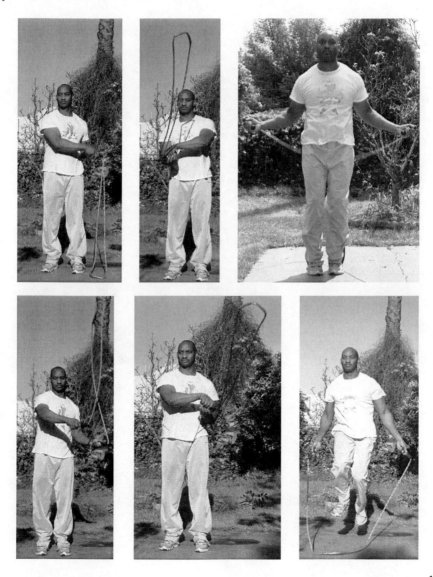

JUMP ROPE EXERCISES

Basic Jump Rope

Beginning Position:
Start while standing with your feet together and the jump rope in both hands.

Action:
Rotate the rope around your body and jump over the rope to complete your reps

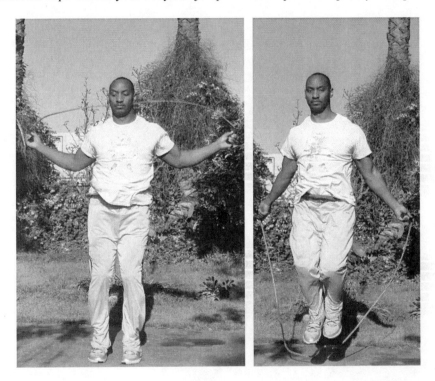

Reverse Jump Rope

Beginning Position:
Start while standing with your feet together and the jump rope in both hands.
Place the rope in front of your feet and body.

Action:
Begin jumping and rotating the rope from the front of your body to the back of your body. Jump before the rope meets your heels to complete your reps.

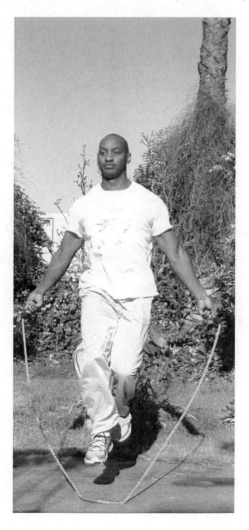

JUMP ROPE EXERCISES

Alternating Footstep

Beginning Position:
Start while keeping your feet close together.

Action:
Alternate your foot strikes as you jump side to side like a boxer.

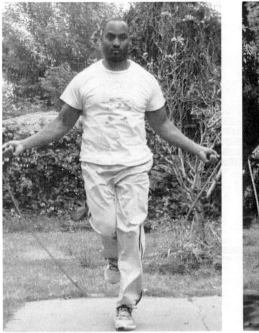
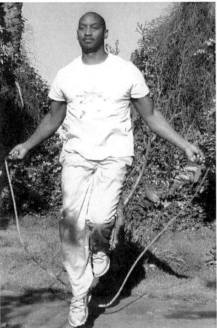

Jog/Run

Beginning Position:
Start while jumping through the turning rope.

Action:
Jog in place. To run, increase your foot and rope speed as you jog or run in place.

Optional:
Jog or run through the rope for a selected distance.

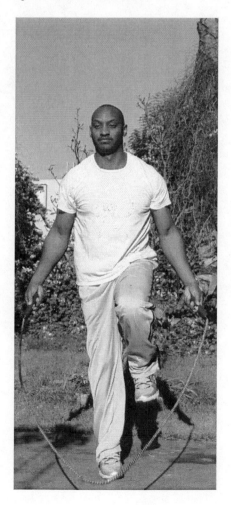

JUMP ROPE EXERCISES

Skier

Beginning Position:
Stand with your feet close together and your knees bent.

Action:
Jump from side to side as you mimic the skiing movements.

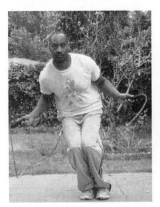 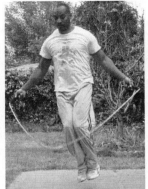 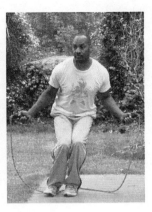

JUMP ROPE EXERCISES

Twist

Beginning Position:
Start while keeping your feet together.

Action:
As you jump rope, jump and twist at the waist in the air, landing with your knees bent as you rotate from side to side.

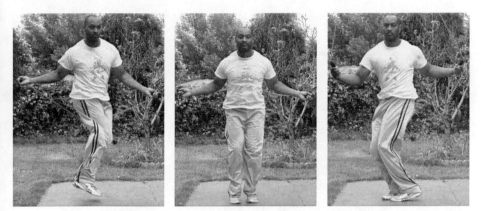

JUMP ROPE EXERCISES

Jackhammer

Beginning Position:
Jump rope while in a half-squat position.

Action:
Rapidly tap your feet on the ground as many times as you can before the rope returns to your feet. When the rope returns to your feet, jump over the rope with both feet to complete your reps.

Optional:
When the rope returns to your feet, jump over the rope with one foot and alternate your feet between each jackhammer.

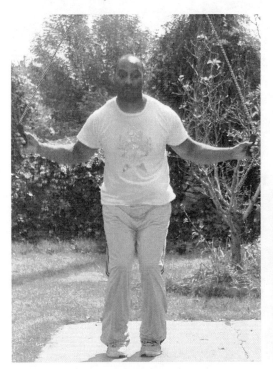
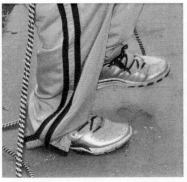

JUMP ROPE EXERCISES

High Knee

Beginning Position:
Start while jumping rope.

Action:
Raise your knees past your belly button or above without bending your back.

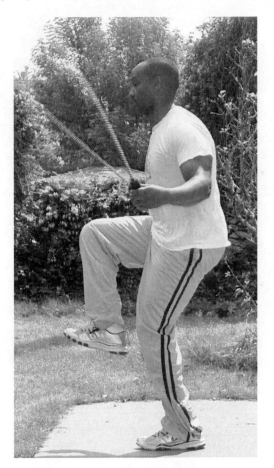

JUMP ROPE EXERCISES

Squat Jump

Beginning Position:
Start while standing in the squatting position.

Action:
Begin jumping and keeping your hips in the flexed position. Try not to stand straight up as you complete your set.

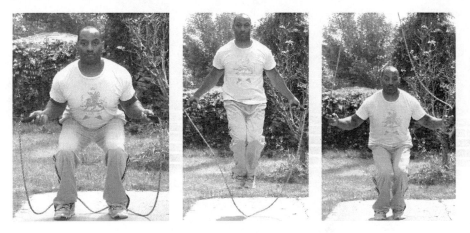

JUMP ROPE EXERCISES

Wave Squat Jump Rope

Beginning Position:
Start while standing with your knees bent and keeping your back flat.

Action:
Start jumping. Upon landing, land with your knees bent on the first jump.
On the second jump, land in the quarter-squat position.
On the third jump, land in the half-squat position
On the fourth jump, perform a double under and land in the full squat position. Repeat
to complete your set.

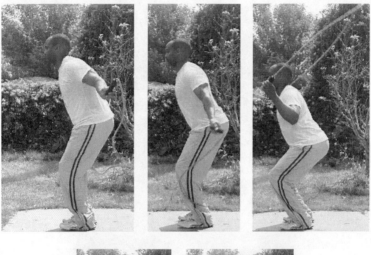

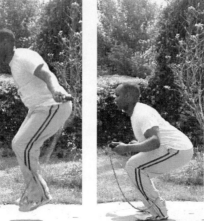

JUMP ROPE EXERCISES

Double Under

Beginning Position:
Jump rope with your feet hip-width apart.

Action:
As the rope rotates around your body, jump higher to allow the rope to pass under your feet two times before your land. Repeat the exercise to complete your reps.

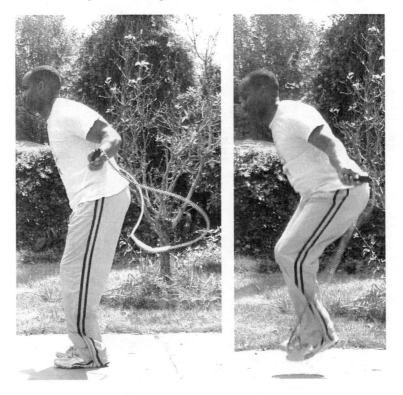

Rope Crossovers

Beginning Position:
Jump rope with your feet together.

Action:
As the rope rotates around your body, cross your arms when the rope is directly above your head. Pull your arms apart to the basic jump rope position before the rope hits the ground. Repeat the exercise to complete your set.

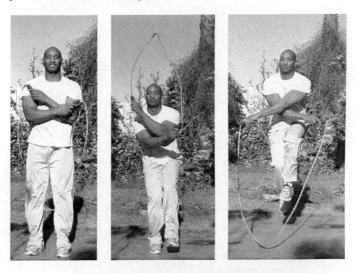

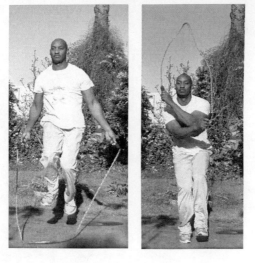

JUMP ROPE EXERCISES

Leg Crossover Jumps

Beginning Position:
Jump rope with your feet together.

Action:
Cross your legs by placing one leg in front of the other leg. Bring your legs apart while jumping and cross the other leg in front to alternate your leg crossing. Continue the leg-cross jumping until you complete your set.

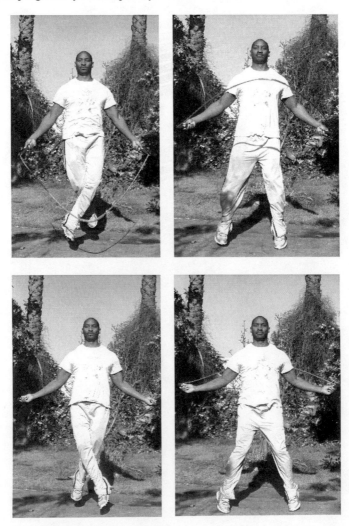

Reverse Rope Crossovers

Beginning Position:
Place the rope in front of your feet and body and jump rope with your feet together.

Action:
Begin jumping and rotating the rope from the front of your body to the back of your body.

As the rope rotates around your body, cross your arms when the rope is directly above your head.

Pull your arms apart to the basic jump rope position before the rope can hit your heels.

Repeat the exercise to complete your reps.

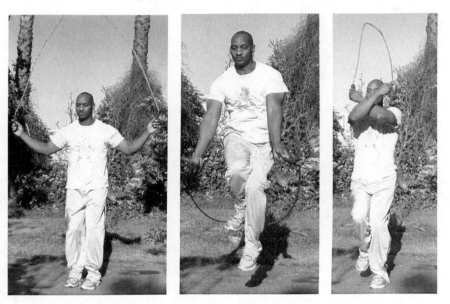

Chapter 5

THE BENEFITS OF SANDBAG TRAINING

During my short twelve years of working with clients, I've found that most people want results, and they want them now. For this fact, I'm providing a brief overview as to why sandbags are of great benefit as a training tool. Following the overview will be the exercises and programs you have been waiting for.

Simply put, the benefit of training with sandbags is the variety. They are highly interchangeable with dumbbell, barbell exercises, and other similar weight lifting modalities. If you can perform a power clean with a barbell, you might try power cleaning a sandbag to add a change in your routine.

The results of training with sandbags will vary based on your form and how you use them to achieve your goals. When working-out with sandbags, in terms of using the correct form, sandbag exercises allow room for imperfect form. As the sand in the bags move, you also have to move and make adjustments with your form, which will alter your technique.

The added movements of the sandbags will cause more healthy stress on your central nervous system. Although the power transfer from using the sandbag differs from using dumbbells or barbells, the functionality of the sandbag is equal if not better.

As I promised I would be brief. I will close the chapter by introducing the exercises along with a few routines for you to enjoy.

Chapter 6

SANDBAG EXERCISES

SANDBAG CORE EXERCISES

Snatch

Beginning Position:
Start with your body in the deadlift position.

Action:
Slowly stand up. As the bag approaches your knees, jump upward to shrug and pull the sandbag over your head. To catch the bag, bend your knees and lock your arms at the elbow.

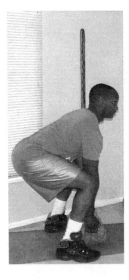 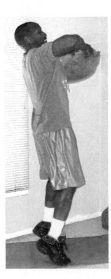 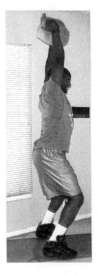

SANDBAG CORE EXERCISES

Snatch, Toss, and Catch

Beginning Position:
Stand in the beginning snatch position.

Action:
Perform a sandbag snatch. As the sandbag approaches your chest, continue to pull the bag. Release the bag when the bag and your arms are over your head. Bend your knees to catch the sandbag as it comes down. Lower the bag to the floor to reposition yourself for more reps.

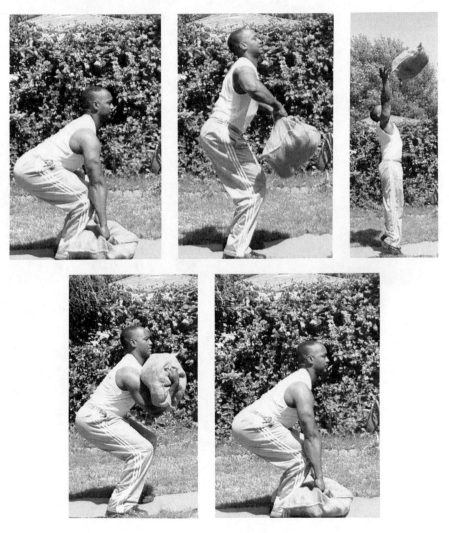

SANDBAG CORE EXERCISES

Power Clean

Beginning Position:
Start while in a squatting position with your feet slightly wider than hip-width apart to allow clearance for the sandbag.

Action:
Grab the sandbag with both hands and explosively stand straight up to pull the sandbag to your chest. Tuck your arm under the sandbag to catch it when it is at or above your chest. Remember to bend your knees to absorb the catch.

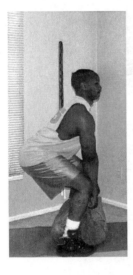 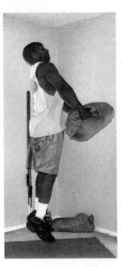 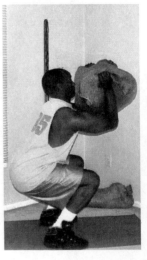

SANDBAG CORE EXERCISES

Up Down/Burpee Power Clean

Beginning Position:
Start with your feet shoulder-width apart to allow clearance for the sandbag.

Action:
Drop down to perform an up down/burpee. Land with both hands on the sandbag. Hop into the starting power clean position and power clean the sandbag.

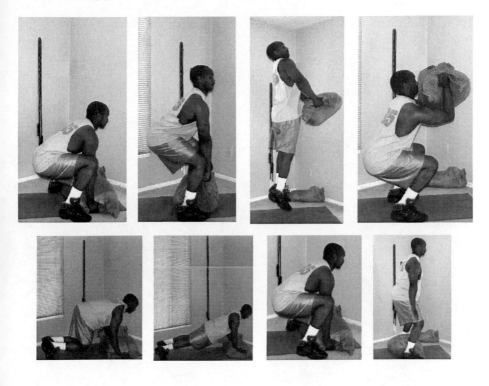

SANDBAG CORE EXERCISES

Overhead Squat

Beginning Position:

Start while in a squat position with your feet slightly wider than your shoulder width. Hold the sandbag over your head with your arms straight and locked at the elbow.

Action:
Maintain straight arms with your chest up and squat down and stand up.

Notes:
Keep your head straight and aligned with your spine.
Keep your arms aligned with your ears.

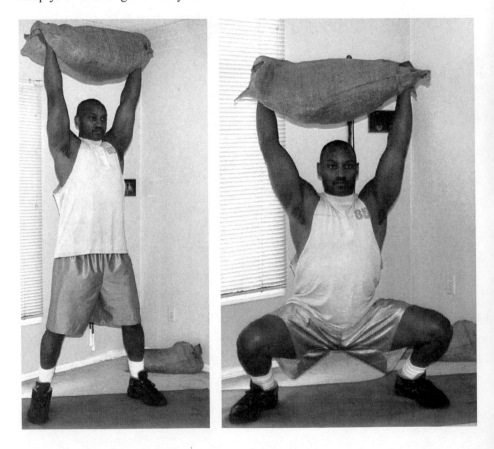

SANDBAG CORE EXERCISES

Squat Press

Beginning Position:
Start with your feet wider than hip width and sandbags at your shoulders,

Action:
Squat down and hold the position to perform a shoulder press. After you press the sandbags, return the sandbags to your shoulders and stand up.

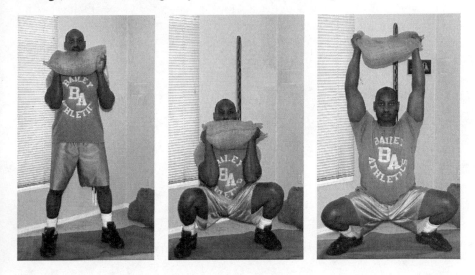

SANDBAG CORE EXERCISES

Overhead Shifting Squat

Beginning Position:
Start while in a wide stance, placing your feet slightly wider than shoulder width. Keep your arms straight up over your head and locked at the elbow.

Action:
As you squat down, shift your body weight to your left or right side. While squatting shift the sandbag over your head and away from your squatting leg. After you reach a ninety-degree flexion at your knees and hips, remain in the squat position and shift your body weight and sandbag to their other side.

Complete the movement by returning the sandbag and body weight to the center of your body and stand up.

Notes:
Keep your head up.

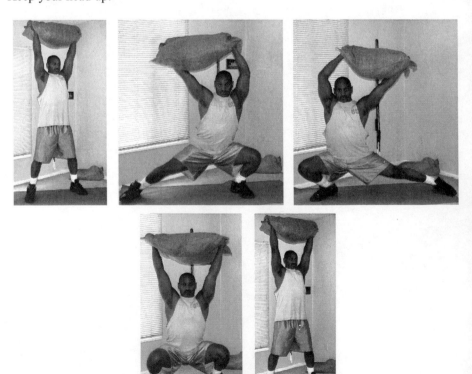

SANDBAG CORE EXERCISES

Side-to-side Overhead Squat

Beginning Position:
Start while in a wide stance, placing your feet slightly wider than shoulder width. Keep your arms straight up over your head.

Action:
Squat down and shift your body to your left or right side. Perform a full squat. Remain in the squatting position and shift your body to the other side. Keep your arms straight and over your head. Complete to movement by returning to the center of your body and stand up. Keep your head aligned with your spine.

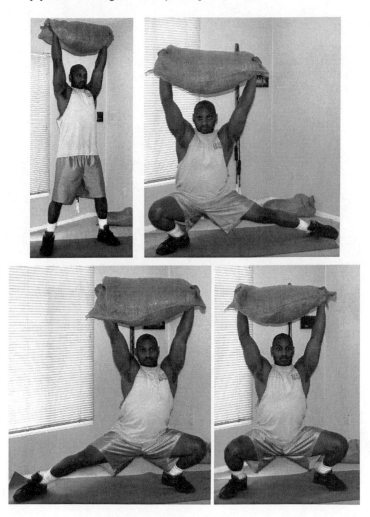

Sandbag Core Exercises

Front Squat

Beginning Position:
Start while standing with your feet shoulder-width apart and holding the sandbag in both hands at your shoulder.

Action:
Squat down until your legs are parallel to the floor.

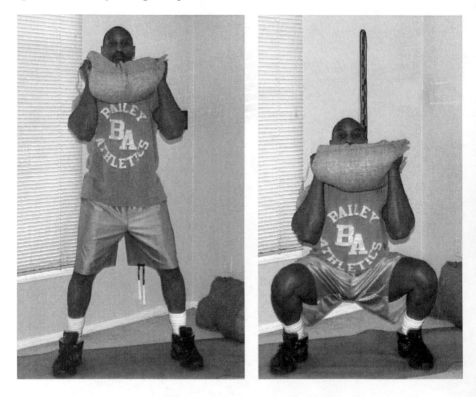

SANDBAG CORE EXERCISES

Swings

Beginning Position:
Start while standing in a squatting position with both of your hands on the sandbag.

Action:
Forcefully stand up and extend your hips and knees to accelerate the sandbag.

Optional:
Use one hand to perform the swing.

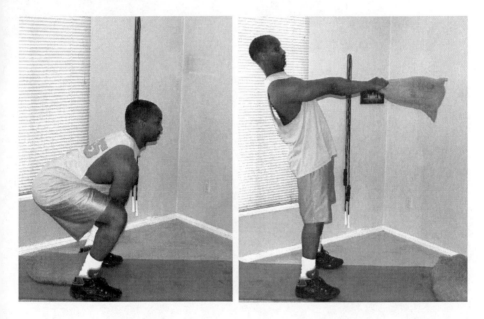

SANDBAG CORE EXERCISES

Front Rack Crossover Lunge

Beginning Position:
Start while standing with the sandbags in your hands and over your shoulders.

Action:
Place your feet hip-width apart. Perform a crossover lunge. Return to the starting position to complete your reps.

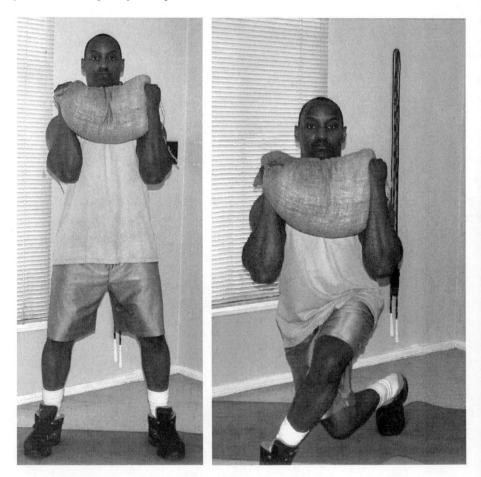

SANDBAG CORE EXERCISES

Front Lunge

Beginning Position:
Hold the sandbags at your shoulders.

Action:
Step forward to perform a lunge.

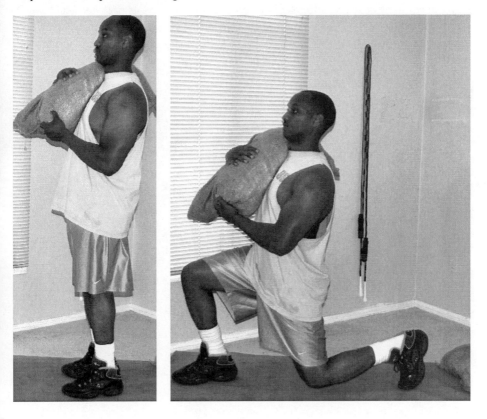

SANDBAG CORE EXERCISES

Round Back Squat

Beginning Position:
Start with your feet wide enough to stand over the sandbag.

Action:
Squat down until your chest touches the sandbag to cause your back to round. Shift your body weight to your heels. Tighten your abs to slowly use your legs, stand up, and straighten your posture. Pause with a slight extension in your hips.

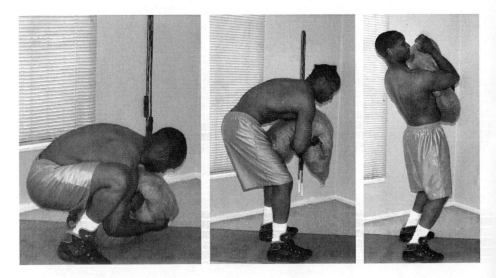

SANDBAG CORE EXERCISES

Shouldering

Beginning Position:
Start while standing in a squatting position with your feet shoulder-width apart to allow clearance for the sandbag.

Action:
Place the sandbag between your feet. Grab the sandbag with both hands and lay it over your shoulder.

Note:
Be sure to use both sides for this exercise.

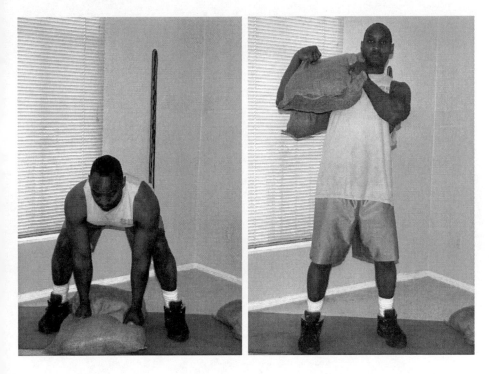

SANDBAG CORE EXERCISES

Diagonal Shouldering

Beginning Position:
Start while in a bottom squatting position with the sandbag on your left or right side.

Action:
Grab the sandbag and stand up to lay the sandbag on the opposite shoulder of your starting position.

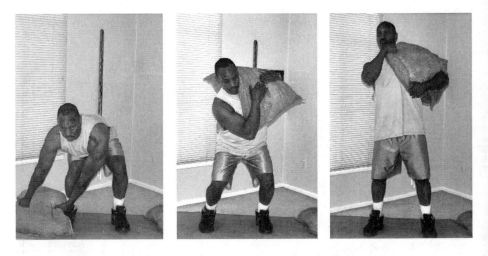

Sᴀɴᴅʙᴀɢ Cᴏʀᴇ Exᴇʀᴄɪsᴇs

Push Press

Beginning Position:
Start while standing with your feet shoulder-width apart.

Action:
Bend your knees and stand up using a thrusting motion to gain momentum and press the sandbag up and over your head.

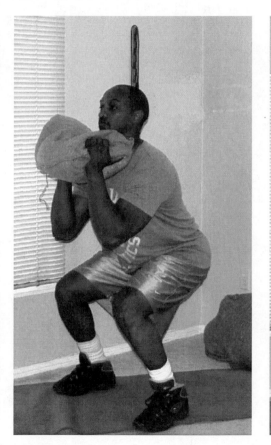
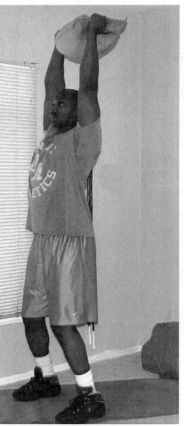

SANDBAG CORE EXERCISES

Side Press

Beginning Position:
Start while standing with your feet shoulder-width apart and staggered.

Action:
Bend the knee of your front leg. With the sandbag in the same hand of your back leg, bend to your side while keeping the sandbag close to your shoulder and press the bag toward the sky. Return the bag to your shoulder and stand up to complete the movement.

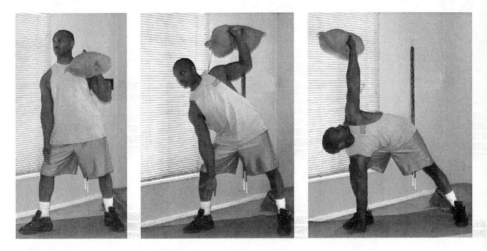

UPPER BODY PUSHING EXERCISES

UPPER BODY PUSHING SANDBAG EXERCISES

Neider Press

Beginning Position:
With your knees bent and feet hip-width apart, hold the sandbags at your shoulders as your elbows point toward the ground.

Action:
Push the sandbag out and away horizontally. Keep the bag above the base of your neck. Return to your starting position to complete your reps.

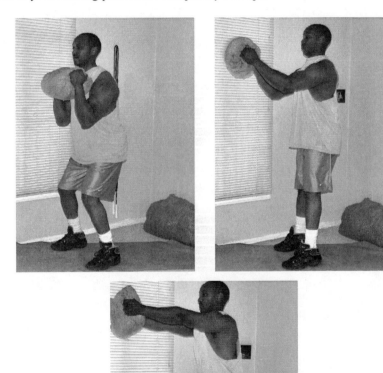

UPPER BODY PUSHING SANDBAG EXERCISES

Shoulder Press

Beginning Position:
Start while standing with your feet shoulder-width apart.

Action:
Keep your legs locked and press the sandbag over your head using your arms and your shoulders.

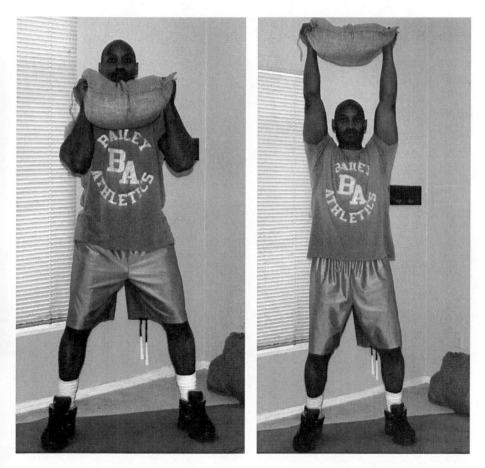

Upper Body Pulling Sandbag Exercises

UPPER BODY PULLING SANDBAG EXERCISES

Bent-over Row

Beginning Position:
Start with your feet shoulder-width apart.

Action:
Bend your knees and lower your shoulders. Your back should be straight and at a forty-five-degree angle. Hold the sandbag in both hands and pull the sandbag to your chest.

Optional:
Use one hand.

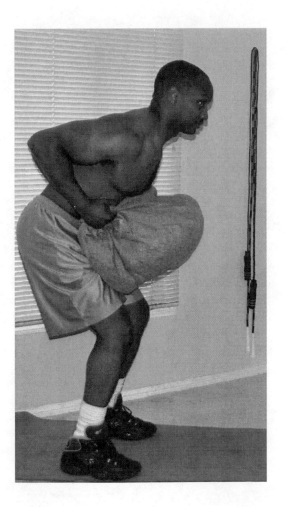

UPPER BODY PUSHING SANDBAG EXERCISES

Round Back Bent-over Row

Beginning Position:
Start with your feet hip-width apart and the sandbag in both hands. Your legs slightly bent.

Action:
Lower your upper body by bending over with a round back. Straighten your back while holding the sandbags. When you are in the classic bent-over row position, perform one rowing repetition and return to the starting position to complete more reps.

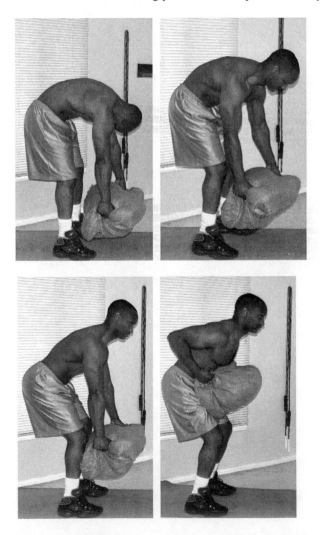

Bicep Curls

Beginning Position:
Stand with your feet shoulder-width apart. Grab the sandbag in one or both hands.

Action:
Curl the sandbag until your arm has reached its full range of motion.

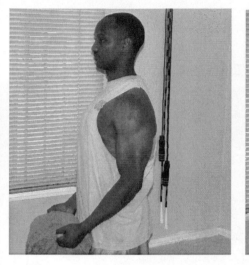 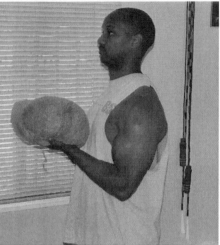

Lower Body Sandbag Exercises

LOWER BODY SANDBAG EXERCISES

Deadlift

Beginning Position:
Start squatting with your feet wider than shoulder-width apart to allow room for your sandbag.

Action:
Keep your chest up, your butt lower than your shoulders and your back flat. Look straight ahead as you push off your heels and stand up.

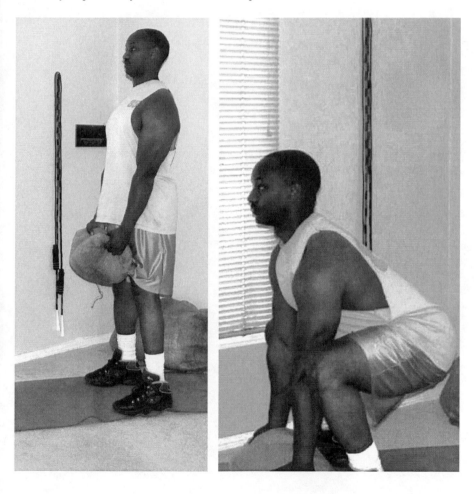

LOWER BODY SANDBAG EXERCISES

Romanian Deadlift

Beginning Position:
Stand straight up with your feet hip-width apart. Hold the sandbag in both hands.

Action:
While keeping your back flat, slightly bend your knees about fifteen to twenty degrees flexion. Hold your legs in the bent position and lower your shoulders by bending at your hips until you feel a stretch in your hamstrings.

Return to the starting position and complete the reps.

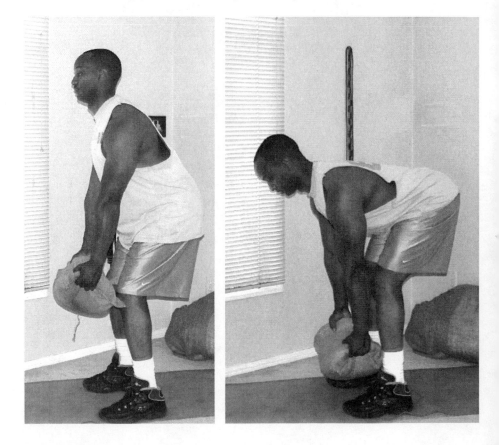

LOWER BODY SANDBAG EXERCISES

Lateral Lunge

Beginning Position:
Stand with your feet hip-width apart and holding the sandbag in front of you with both hands.

Action:
Step out to your side with one leg and bend your knee. Try to keep the knee of your support leg over your big toe.

Optional:
Hold the sandbag on your shoulder or over your back.

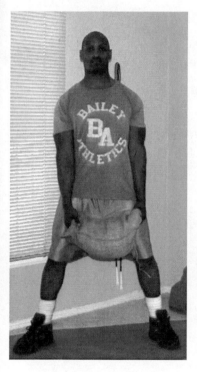 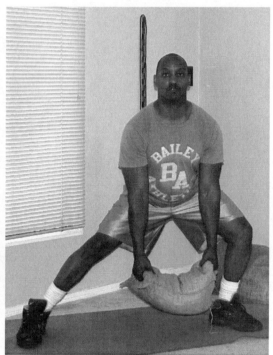

Chapter 7

Body Weight Exercise Routine

General Fitness

Complete this one time in thirty minutes or less or two times in one hour or less.		
Exercises	**Reps**	**Rest**
Dive bomber	16	keep going
Sea saw planks	20 each side	keep going
Clapping push-up or compression push-ups	12	keep going
Single-leg jackknife	10 each side	keep going
Stride crunches	12 each side	keep going
Pull-ups	15	keep going
Bicycle crunches	20 each side	keep going
Squat kick-outs	20	keep going
Half push-up, come up, and dive bomber = one rep	16	keep going
Tuck jumps	15	keep going
Side-to-side pull-ups	4 each side	keep going
Incline wide push-up	12	keep going
Rocking Crunch	45-60 sec	keep going
Tuck jumps	16	keep going

Diamond push-ups	15	keep going
Superman	20	keep going
Pull-ups	15	keep going
3-D up down/burpee	6	keep going
Deep sumo squat walk	32 steps	keep going
Rest 90 seconds		

Full-body Core Circuit

Split Jump lunges with bat arm swing motion—4 each side
Up down—6
Side plank "left or right"—10
Horizontal Row—6
Full-body or Modified bridge—6
Rocking crunch—10
Woodchopper—6
Time Clock—6
Side plank other side—10

General Fitness 2

Exercises		Reps	
Side-to-side push-up		10	
Horizontal pull-ups		10	
Kick-out squats		10	each side
Pull-ups		10	
Broad jumps		10	

Rest 1 minute　　　　　　　　　**Repeat 2 more times**

Exercises		Reps	
Body rolling		20	10 left 10 right
Circle pull-ups		16	8 left 8 right
Woodchopper		15	
Dive bombers		15	
Duck walk		15	

Rest 1minute　　　　　　　　　**Repeat 2 more times**

Exercises		Reps	
Grasshopper up downs		20	
Standing windmill		20	
Acceleration/deceleration lunge		20	
Wide grip pull-ups		20	
One leg supported squat jump		20	10 each side

Rest 1minute　　　　　　　　　**Repeat 2 more times**

Ab Circuit		Reps	Rest
Jackknife		10	0
Windshield wiper		10	0
Seesaw plank		20	0
Half jackknifes		10	0
Medial side plank		30 sec	0
Bicycle crunches		10	0

Seated leg lifts		10	0
Single-leg incline plank, one side only		30 sec	0
Sit-ups		10	0
Single-leg jackknife, slow on the way down		10	0
Standing windmill		10	0
Single-leg incline plank other side		30 sec	0
6 minute Interval		time set	rest
Tuck jumps		30 sec	15 sec
Hand walking		30 sec	15 sec
Ice skater		30 sec	15 sec
Up down with pull-ups*		30 sec	15 sec
Wall squats		30 sec	15 sec
3-D plank jump		30 sec	15 sec

*Repeat the sequence under a pull-up bar, one up down then two pull-ups.

Optional: add a weight vest after the first round.

Twenty-Minute Morning or Evening

Exercises	Sets and Repetitions		Rest
Side-to-side push-up	3	each side	25 sec
3-D Squat and tap	5		25 sec
Modified horizontal row	6		25 sec
Dive bombers	3		25 sec
Squats	3		25 sec
Single-leg bridges	3	each side	25 sec
Horizontal row	3		25 sec
Lateral lunge	5	each side	25 sec
Woodchopper	8		25 sec
Crunches	10		25 sec

Repeat for up to twenty minutes.

Explosive Multi-planar Leg Workout

Exercises	Sets and Repetitions	Rest
Woodchoppers	1x10+ 1x15 + 2x10	30 sec rest
Wall squat	2x10-5-second holds	30 sec rest
Sumo squat walk	3-4x10	30 sec rest
Ice skater	3x6	45 sec rest
Jumping jack squats	4x6	45 sec rest
Lateral frog jumps	4x10	45 sec rest
Wall squat	1x10-5-second holds	30 sec rest
Jumping jack squats	1x10 + 1x6 1x10	45 sec rest
2-minute rest		
Medial Side Plank	3x12	30 sec rest
Superman	4x15	30 sec rest
Bicycle crunches	2x40	30 sec rest
Jackknife	5x10	30 sec rest

Pre-weight Conditioning

Exercises	Sets and Reps						
Clapping push-up	5	6	5	6	5	6	5
Bear crawl backwards	5 yards	6 yards	5 yards	6 yards	5 yards	6 yards	5 yards
Clapping push-up	5	6	5	6	5	6	5
Single-leg wall squats	15-40 sec	16-40 sec	15-40 sec	16-40 sec	15-40 sec	16-40 sec	15-40 sec
Rocking crunches	30	30	30	30	30	30	30
Jackknife	20	20	20	20	20	20	20
Chin-ups	10	10	10	10	10	10	10
Full-body bridge	12	12	12	12	12	12	12
Double under jump rope	20	25	30	20	25	30	32
Crossover lunge	8+8	12+12	15+15	12+12	10+10	15+15	12+12
Woodchopper	12	12	12	12	12	12	12

with 1-4 lbs heavy rope

Note:

For circuit training starting from top to bottom.

Ten-Minute Abs Routine   With or Without Sandbags

Exercises	Repetitions	Rest
Time clock	20	30
Seated leg lifts	15	30
Rocking bicycle crunches	24	30
Jackknifes or supported JK	10	30
Elbow bridge	30 sec	30
Side planks	12 each	30
Time clock	16	30
Bent knee hip lifts	12	30
Sit-ups	30	30

Repeat for ten minutes or perform each exercise for
forty-five seconds and rest thirty seconds
between sets.

Posterior Muscle Development

Exercises	Sets and Repetitions		
Wide jumping jack squats	2-5 sets	10 reps	
Crossover lunge	2-5 sets	8 reps	each side
Up-downs	2-5 sets	8 reps	
Single-leg bridge	2-5 sets	8 reps	each side
Acceleration/Deceleration lunge	2-5 sets	8 reps	each side
Seesaw plank	2-5 sets	16 reps	
Woodchopper	2-5 sets	8 reps	
Standing windmill	2-5 sets	16 reps	
Dive bomber push-ups	2-5 sets	8 reps	
Elbow bridge	2-5 sets	20 sec	

Use a sandbag if or when the routine is too easy.

Circular Core Routine   Perform 3-4 sets

Exercises	Reps	weight
Standing windmill	10	
Windshield wiper	20	
Grasshopper burpee	6	
Circular pull-ups	20	
Circular push-ups	20	
Acceleration/deceleration lunge	10	each side
Sandbag swings	20	sandbag
Standing windmill	10	

Fifteen-Minute Lateral Body Weight Routine

Exercise	Reps
Lateral Frog Jumps	15
3-D Up Downs	15
Ice Skater	15
Side Plank w/ Hip tap*	15
Seated leg lifts	15
Crossover Push-Ups	15
Side-to-Side Pull-Ups	15
Woodchoppers	15
Windshield Wipers	15

Repeat for fifteen minutes.

* Tap your hip on the mat

Volleyball

Exercises	Sets and Reps	Rest	Weight
Sumo squat and reach	10	25 sec rest	w/ sandbag
Up downs	6	25 sec rest	
Jumping pull-up	15	25 sec rest	
Hand walk	10	25 sec rest	
Up downs (with backboard tap; optional)	6	25 sec rest	
Horizontal row	10	25 sec rest	
Single-leg wall squat	30 sec	w/o rest	
Bicycle crunches	40	30 sec rest	
Woodchopper	1x10 + 1x15 + 2x10	40 sec rest	w/ sandbag
Wall squat	2x10 (5-second holds)	40 sec rest	w/ sandbag
Ice skater	3x12	40 sec rest	w/ sandbag
Sumo squat walk	3x10	40 sec rest	w/ sandbag
Jumping jack squats	4x6	40 sec rest	w/ sandbag
Single-leg wall squat	1set of 10 (5-second holds)	40 sec rest	w/ sandbag
Lateral frog jumps = zigzag	1x10 + 1x6 + 1x10	40 sec rest	w/ sandbag
2-minute rest			
Elevated medial side plank	3x25 sec each side	30 sec rest	
Superman	4x15	30 sec rest	
Bicycle crunches	2x40	30 sec rest	
Jackknife	5x10	30 sec rest	

Tennis and Basketball

You can perform these routine in two ways.

Exercises	↓→ Sets and Repetitions				Rest
Standing windmill	12	12	12	12	30 sec
Lateral frog jump	6	6	6	6	30 sec
Deep sumo squats	10	10	10	10	30 sec
Windshield wiper	20	20	20	20	30 sec
Side-to-side push-ups plus clapping push-ups	4 + 12	4 + 12	4 + 12	4 + 12	30 sec
Bicep Blaster	12	12	12	12	30 sec
One leg supported jump squat	8	8	8	8	30 sec
Wide grip pull-ups	10	10	10	10	30 sec
Compression push-ups	10	10	10	10	30 sec
Lateral frog jump	12	16	20	20	30 sec
Handstand Pushup	6	6	6	6	30 sec
Superman	15	15	15	15	30 sec

Senior Workout

Exercises	Sets and Repetitions		Rest
Modified push-ups	10		30 sec
Wall squats	30 sec		30 sec
Sea saw planks	20		30 sec
Push-ups	10		30 sec
Lateral lunges	16	each side	30 sec
Modified horizontal row	12		30 sec
Single-leg bridges	10	each side	30 sec
Bicycle crunches	20		30 sec
Modified horizontal row	15		30 sec

Repeat for 45-60 min

Chapter 8

JUMP ROPE ROUTINES

To enhance the sample jump rope workouts, use guidelines listed below.

1. Select an intensity method. Try the heart rate method or the rotations per minute (rpm) method. See the chart.
2. Choose the jump rope exercises that helps you reach your athletic fitness goal, (e.g., timing, agility, coordination.
3. Choose the jump rope exercises that are suitable for your athletic fitness level. (e.g., ankle, hip, spine, shin tolerance, cardio tolerance.
4. Use low rpm's to learn a new jump rope technique. Try to use transition jump rope exercises instead of stopping.
5. Work hard, have fun, and get in shape!

Slow Pace—Used for learning new techniques, warm-up, cooling down, transitions

65 percent - 70 percent heart rate or 135 rotations per minute or less

Medium Pace—Used for warm-up, aerobic conditioning, transitions

75 percent - 85 percent heart rate or 135-159 rotations per minute

Fast Pace—Used for anaerobic conditioning and transitions

85 percent - 95 percent plus heart rate or 160 rotations per minute or more

Average Target Heart Rate Percentage Chart

Age Groups	65%	70%	75%	80%	85%	90%	95%
15-19	132	141	151	161	172	182	192
20-29	127	137	147	156	166	176	186
30-39	121	130	140	148	158	167	176
40-49	114	123	133	140	149	158	167
50-59	108	116	125	132	141	149	157

Five-Day Jump Rope Strength and Conditioning Sample Program

Monday	Tuesday	Wednesday	Thursday	Friday	Saturday	Sunday
Warm up 5-7 min	Warm up 5-7 min	Warm up 5-7 min	Warm up 5-7 min	Warm up 5-7 min		
Jump rope interval training 30 min	Jump rope speed development routine day 1	Jump rope speed development routine day 1 or 2	Active rest	Jump rope interval training 20-25 min	Off Day	Off Day
		Rest 3-5 min				
Abs and upper body weight exercises		General conditioning body weight program 1		Abs and lower body sandbag exercises		

Jump Rope Speed Development

Alternate your sets with a heavy rope and a speed rope.

Heavy Rope—weight 1-4 lbs

Slow-paced warm-up
5-8 minutes with light rope

Day 1	Medium Pace or 75%-85% HR	Time	Rest
Set 1	Heavy Rope	20 sec	75 sec
Set 2	Speed Rope	25 sec	90 sec
Set 3	Heavy Rope	30 sec	110 sec
Set 4	Speed Rope	25 sec	90 sec
Set 5	Heavy Rope	30 sec	110 sec
Set 6	Speed Rope	25 sec	90 sec
Set 7	Heavy Rope	15 sec	55 sec
Set 8	Speed Rope	10 sec	35 sec
Set 9	Speed Rope	15 sec	55 sec
Day 2	Medium-Fast Pace or 85%-95% + HR	Time	Rest
Set 1	Heavy Rope	15 sec	45 sec
Set 2	Speed Rope	20 sec	65 sec
Set 3	Heavy Rope	30 sec	95 sec
Set 4	Speed Rope	25 sec	80 sec
Set 5	Speed Rope	30 sec	95 sec
Set 6	Heavy Rope	25 sec	80 sec
Set 7	Speed Rope	15 sec	45 sec
Set 8	Speed Rope	10 sec	35 sec
Set 9	Heavy Rope	10 sec	35 sec
Set 10	Speed Rope	15 sec	45 sec
Set 11	Heavy Rope	15 sec	50 sec
Set 12	Speed Rope	15 sec	50 sec
Set 13	Speed Rope	10 sec	35 sec
Set 14	Speed Rope	15 sec	45 sec

1-2-3 Jump Rope Agility Routine

1

Jump one time forward on both feet.

Jump one time backward on both feet.

Jump two times forward on both feet.

Jump two times backward on both feet.

Jump three times forward on both feet.

Jump three times backward on both feet.

2

Jump one time forward on one foot.

Jump one time backward on one foot.

Plant both feet.

Jump two times forward on one foot.

Jump two times backward on one foot.

Plant both feet.

Jump three times forward on one foot.

Jump three times backward on one foot.

Repeat on your other leg.

3

Jump and land one time on one foot forward.

Jump one time backward on the same foot.

Land and plant both feet.

Jump and land one time on your other foot forward

Jump one time backward on the same foot.

Land and plant both feet.

Jump and land two times on one foot forward,

Jump backward on the same foot.

Land and plant on both feet.

Jump two times backward on both feet.

Jump and land two times on your other foot forward.

Jump backward on the same foot

Land and plant both feet.

Jump two times backward on both feet—do not pause.

Jump and land three times on one foot forward.

Jump backward on the same foot.

Land and plant both feet.

Jump and land three times on your other foot forward.

Jump backward on the same foot.

Land and plant both feet.

Jump three times backward on both feet.

Third step can be started by jumping either forward or backward.

Chapter 9

SANDBAG EXERCISE ROUTINES

Sandbag Routine		
Exercises	Repetitions	Sets
Sandbag Side to side overhead squats	6	3-5
Sandbag cleans	6	3-5
Sandbag step-through lunge	8-10	3-5
Sandbag round back squats	6	3-5
Sandbag neider press	8	3-5
Sandbag push press	8	3-5
Sandbag bent over row	10	3-5
Sandbag squat press	6	3-5
Sandbag bicep curls	10	3-5
Sandbag swings	8	3-5
Sandbag side press	5 each side	3-5

BA - 8

Exercises	Repetitions	Sets	Rest
Sandbag snatch—side to side shifting squat	8	8	40 sec max
Sandbag bicep curls—neider press—bent over row	1 each 8x	8	40 sec max
Sandbag lateral lunge—crossover lunge—shouldering	8/8/8	8	40 sec max
Sandbag Swings	8	8	40 sec max
Sandbag updown clean	8	8	40 sec max
Sandbag diagonal shouldering—push press	8	8	40 sec max
Sandbag front squats	8	8	40 sec max
Sandbag toss & catch with updown	8	8	40 sec max

Chapter 10

COMBINATION EXERCISE ROUTINES

Body Weight Jump Rope Routine

Exercises		Reps	Rest
Broad jump plus double under		3 + 6	30 sec
Lateral up downs		8	30 sec
Jackknife fast on the way up, slow on the way down		6	30 sec
Pull-ups		10	30 sec
One leg jump rope for height		5/5	30 sec
Circle push-up		5R5L	30 sec
Bicep blaster		8	30 sec
Broad jump plus double under		3 + 6	45 sec
Lateral up downs		8	30 sec
Jackknife fast on the way up, slow on the way down		12	30 sec
Pull-up		8	30 sec
Ice skater jump rope		2 min	30 sec
Clapping push-up		10	30 sec
Bicep blaster pull-up		8	30 sec
Double under		25	60 sec

Jackknife fast on the way up, slow on the way down		20	30 sec
Time clock up downs		8	15 sec
Side-to-side pull-up		8	30 sec
Speed jump rope		20 sec	30 sec
Circle push-up		5R5L	30 sec
Duck walk		10 steps	30 sec

Sandbag BWT Circuit 1

Exercises		Reps
3-D plank jump		5
Grasshopper burpee		5
Sandbag overhead squat		5
Push press		3
Upright row		3
Swing plus snatch to throw and catch		6 + 6
Woodchopper		10

Repeat six times.

Sandbag Jump Rope BWT Routine 1

**Medium Pace or
75%-85% HR**

Jump Rope Style and Time			Exercises	Reps	Rest
Jackhammer	105 sec	→	Up down	5	45 sec
Reverse jump rope	110 sec	→	SB upright row	12	30 sec
Leg crossovers	115 sec	→	Up down	5	1 min
Rope crossovers	130 sec	→	SB round back squat	10	2 min
Jump rope	120 sec	→	Medial side plank	30 sec each	30 sec
Jackhammer	1 min	→	Pull-ups	125 sec	30 sec

Sand Bag Jump Rope BWT Routine 2

Exercises	Reps
Sandbag clean	6
Frog jumps	12
Time clock	20
Up down plus tuck jump	12
Sandbag clean	5
Single-leg elbow bridge	20 sec hold each
Kick-out squats	4 each leg
Compression push-ups	12
Sandbag clean	6
Sandbag pull-ups with leg raises wght between knees	15
Sandbag front squats	8
Sandbag bent-over row	12-15
Sandbag push press	12
Sandbag snatch—same weight as above	5
Sandbag upright row—same weight as above	10
3-D Up downs	16
Seated leg lift	20
Sandbag clean plus broad jumps—snatch weight	5+5
Pull-ups with leg raises	12
Push-ups	20
Pull-ups with leg raises	15
Push-ups	30

Index

T

U

W

For more information on training to become
athletically fit and healthy visit the author at:
WWW.BAILEYATHLETICS.COM

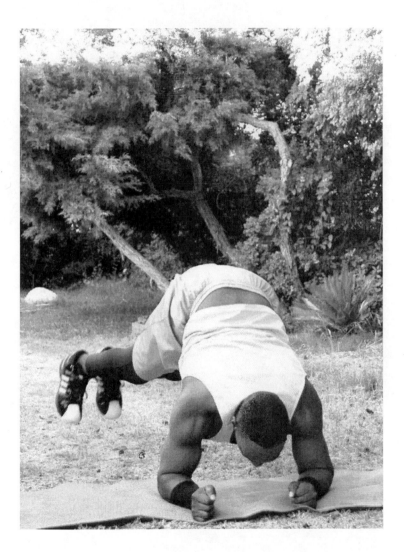